Nuclear Development

ISBN 978-92-64-17637-9



# Nuclear Education and Training: From Concern to Capability


NEA No. 6979

NUCLEAR ENERGY AGENCY
ORGANISATION FOR ECONOMIC CO-OPERATION AND DEVELOPMENT

## ORGANISATION FOR ECONOMIC CO-OPERATION AND DEVELOPMENT

The OECD is a unique forum where the governments of 34 democracies work together to address the economic, social and environmental challenges of globalisation. The OECD is also at the forefront of efforts to understand and to help governments respond to new developments and concerns, such as corporate governance, the information economy and the challenges of an ageing population. The Organisation provides a setting where governments can compare policy experiences, seek answers to common problems, identify good practice and work to co-ordinate domestic and international policies.

The OECD member countries are: Australia, Austria, Belgium, Canada, Chile, the Czech Republic, Denmark, Estonia, Finland, France, Germany, Greece, Hungary, Iceland, Ireland, Israel, Italy, Japan, Luxembourg, Mexico, the Netherlands, New Zealand, Norway, Poland, Portugal, the Republic of Korea, the Slovak Republic, Slovenia, Spain, Sweden, Switzerland, Turkey, the United Kingdom and the United States. The European Commission takes part in the work of the OECD.

OECD Publishing disseminates widely the results of the Organisation's statistics gathering and research on economic, social and environmental issues, as well as the conventions, guidelines and standards agreed by its members.



## NUCLEAR ENERGY AGENCY

The OECD Nuclear Energy Agency (NEA) was established on 1 February 1958. Current NEA membership consists of 30 OECD member countries: Australia, Austria, Belgium, Canada, the Czech Republic, Denmark, Finland, France, Germany, Greece, Hungary, Iceland, Ireland, Italy, Japan, Luxembourg, Mexico, the Netherlands, Norway, Poland, Portugal, the Republic of Korea, the Slovak Republic, Slovenia, Spain, Sweden, Switzerland, Turkey, the United Kingdom and the United States. The European Commission also takes part in the work of the Agency.

The mission of the NEA is:

- to assist its member countries in maintaining and further developing, through international co-operation, the scientific, technological and legal bases required for a safe, environmentally friendly and economical use of nuclear energy for peaceful purposes, as well as
- to provide authoritative assessments and to forge common understandings on key issues, as input to government decisions on nuclear energy policy and to broader OECD policy analyses in areas such as energy and sustainable development.

Specific areas of competence of the NEA include the safety and regulation of nuclear activities, radioactive waste management, radiological protection, nuclear science, economic and technical analyses of the nuclear fuel cycle, nuclear law and liability, and public information.

The NEA Data Bank provides nuclear data and computer program services for participating countries. In these and related tasks, the NEA works in close collaboration with the International Atomic Energy Agency in Vienna, with which it has a Co-operation Agreement, as well as with other international organisations in the nuclear field.



*Cover photos: Training at the* Institut des sciences et techniques nucléaires, *France (L. Godart/CEA, picture provided by I2EN); DELPHI subcritical assembly, the Netherlands (Delft University Technology).*

# Foreword

In 2000, the OECD Nuclear Energy Agency (NEA) published *Nuclear Education and Training: Cause for Concern?*, which, for the first time, drew attention to the likelihood of insufficient human resources being available to support nuclear power plant operations, the decommissioning of existing nuclear facilities and foreseeable developments. Several measures were proposed in the report to encourage urgent intervention by key stakeholders.

Since then, the political and technological landscape has changed considerably with an increased global opportunity for civil nuclear power and expanding demand for a skilled nuclear workforce. Irrespective of changes that may occur in the aftermath of the Fukushima Daiichi accident, significant numbers of highly trained personnel will be required, either in relation to new build or to compensate for the ageing workforce.

This report reviews initiatives that have been undertaken during the last decade by governments, educational and research institutes, and industry, illustrating examples of good practices in a number of countries. Achieving a steady and sustainable supply of workers for the nuclear sector is a challenge not only because of the high numbers involved globally, but also because of the high level of competency required. Concerns remain that sustainable sources of skilled workers have not been established in all areas or in all countries.

As part of the study, a survey was conducted on the use of research facilities and laboratories in NEA member countries for education and training. The results show that, in general, existing infrastructure is underutilised for hands-on education and training, and expensive, unique facilities have been shut down or are due to close over the next few years.

A noteworthy development has been the internationalisation of the nuclear workforce and the associated education and training, partly as a result of globalisation of nuclear technology and its applications, and partly from the recognition that some countries may not have all the facilities needed. This trend puts more emphasis on the need for greater consistency in education and training delivery and course content and, concomitantly, greater need to be able to accredit such training.

Recognising this trend and the overarching priority to ensure safety, and drawing from the experience of a number of countries, the expert group responsible for the study researched and classified a set of job roles with significant nuclear competence found across the nuclear industry. This effort lays the basis for the development of an outline classification system for nuclear job profiles: a job taxonomy framework.

Nuclear job specifications have been produced for the main activities associated with the construction, operation and decommissioning of commercial and research reactors, drawing up on analyses conducted by a number of companies. These may serve as an initial platform on which organisations or governments can overlay their own specific requirements.

The study discusses issues related to the various aspects presented above, identifies areas of outstanding concern and provides a set of recommendations to address them.

## Acknowledgements

This study was carried out under the auspices of the NEA Committee for Technical and Economic Studies on Nuclear Energy Development and the Fuel Cycle and prepared by an ad hoc expert group (see list in Appendix 6) under the chairmanship of Professor Michel Giot. The participation of the expert group members is gratefully acknowledged. Special thanks are due to Brian Murphy for his work on the job taxonomy framework, to Steve Bennett, lead author of Chapter 1, and to Michel Giot, lead author and important contributor of the section on the use of research facilities for education and training.

The involvement of COGENT, TECNATOM, ONET Technologies, OPG, SCK•CEN, ANSTO, CEA and AECL in sourcing and reviewing data for the job taxonomy framework is also gratefully acknowledged, as is the contribution of David Gilchrist who provided a prototype of a job taxonomy application.

The study was supported by NEA Secretariat members Maria Elena Urso, Scientific Secretary for the study, and Ron Cameron, Head of the Nuclear Development Division.

# Table of contents

## Figures



## Tables

# Executive summary

## Background

In 2000, the OECD Nuclear Energy Agency (NEA) published *Nuclear Education and Training: Cause for Concern?*, which, for the first time, drew attention to the likelihood of insufficient human resources being available to support current operations, foreseeable developments and the decommissioning of shut-down nuclear facilities. Several measures were proposed in the report to encourage urgent intervention by key stakeholders. Progress against the recommendations was assessed in 2004 in a follow-up report on *Nuclear Competence Building*. A number of outstanding problems were highlighted, in particular as regards the time required to accumulate sufficient skills and knowledge to achieve competence. The situation was made worse by a loss of existing experience, a contraction in research and training facilities, and reduced university funding. Although greater awareness of the overall future skills deficit had been achieved, it was concluded that the response was geographically variable, and that there had been no breakthrough in addressing the downturn in the skilled nuclear workforce.

Since then, the political and technological landscape has changed considerably with the potential for greater deployment of civil nuclear power driven by increased demand for energy, the need to address climate change, concerns over security of supply, the more attractive economic prospects for nuclear energy in the context of carbon pricing and the desire for long-term stability in energy prices. Such changes bring about a demand for expansion of the skilled nuclear workforce. Furthermore, over the last ten years, nuclear education and training has evolved against a more nuanced understanding of how nuclear skills need to be addressed.

This study assesses the current state of nuclear education and training for the development of nuclear skills, the remaining gaps and the actions that are now required to address corresponding development needs across NEA member countries. Programmes and instruments for human resource development have been analysed in three parts by looking at the provision of specialist nuclear education for nuclear professionals: 1) through a review of initiatives that have been taken over the last ten years by the various actors internationally; 2) through a parallel survey on the use of research facilities for education and training; and 3) through the development of a framework for classifying and typifying a selection of nuclear job profiles.

## The continuing need for human resources

The distinctive characteristics of nuclear energy and its fuel cycle give rise to special requirements for education and training. In all countries with a nuclear programme, even before new build is taken into account and regardless of national policies, there exists a substantial nuclear estate to be safely operated, maintained and in time decommissioned. An essential element in the implementation and safe operation of all nuclear facilities as well as nuclear technology research and development is a knowledgeable and skilled workforce.

The nuclear workforce of the 21$^{st}$ century is a significant international, commercial and research community. Although there is a lack of detailed numerical data at the national and global level, existing surveys conducted in a number of countries suggest that future demand for global employment in nuclear-related activities are in the tens to hundreds of thousands of skilled workers. This is attributable, to a significant extent, to the expected retirement rates of the existing workforce.

A recent study by a Los Alamos National Laboratory team (Li *et al.*, 2009) simulated human resource development needs for several scenarios in the Russian Federation and the United States. Figure E.1 shows the magnitude of the prospective demand for operations personnel (i.e. operating staff retained for plant operations following the construction phase) for the United States case where additional plants are built to retain market share. Starting from the 56 000 United States workforce (as of 2006), the graph shows separately staff needs to replace retiring personnel and to cater for additional capacity, indicating a demand, by 2030, of approximately 19 000 new positions and a total of 63 000 new hires (19 000 + 44 000 to replace retiring employees). The main outcome from this analysis is that there will be a large need for education and training of new employees.

**Figure E.1: Estimates of the operating personnel needed for retaining market share in nuclear power in the United States**

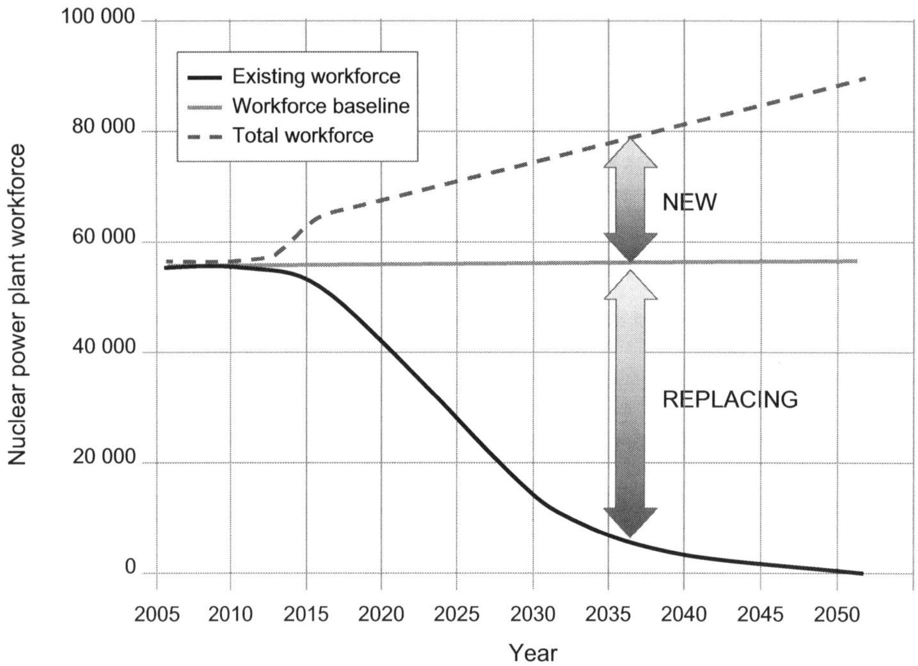


Source: Li *et al.* (2009).

In general, the demand for nuclear skills set against a generally ageing workforce implies that significant intervention will be required to maintain an adequately skilled and competent workforce, and the required flow of new recruits for long-term sustainability. Policy decisions need to be made now to ensure that adequate nuclear education and training infrastructure is available in the decades ahead. Delays and changes in policies will have detrimental effects on sustaining an effective workforce.

Research and development in nuclear technology are increasingly taking place across international borders. Concurrently, civil nuclear deployment and its associated supply chain have undergone internationalisation. As a result, the need has emerged for a more global nuclear workforce.

## A key resource – a competent workforce

The nuclear industry is characterised by a requirement for high overall skill levels and a high degree of safety. Safety is a pre-eminent concern in the nuclear industry not only for its own sake, but also its sensitivity in term of public perception and, formally, because of national and regional regulations and international agreements. The importance of education and training in maintaining safety cannot be understated. For all these reasons, safe behaviours are regarded as critical skills in parallel with the specific technical competencies for the job. Managers and leaders have a key role to model appropriate behaviours and to support nuclear education and training in order to generate and maintain a robust safety culture.

It is useful to recognise that there are various degrees of "nuclearisation" within the industry, that is, the extent to which specific nuclear skills and safety culture training are needed to complement other engineering or management skills. Throughout the workforce, general nuclear awareness is a prerequisite, with more specialised nuclear expertise being required by fewer personnel, depending on the specific job requirements.

A threefold categorisation of the competencies necessary to run a nuclear power plant can be drawn, which includes:

- "nuclear" people with a specialised formal education in nuclear subjects (e.g. nuclear engineering, radiochemistry, radiological protection, etc.);
- "nuclearised" people with formal education and training in a relevant (non-nuclear) area (e.g. mechanical, electrical, civil engineering, systems) but who need to acquire knowledge of the nuclear environment in which they have to apply their competencies;
- "nuclear-aware" people requiring nuclear awareness to work in the industry (e.g. electricians, mechanics, and other crafts and support personnel).

This can be visualised in terms of the pyramid of competence in Figure E.2. Generally there will be a larger number of employees from top to bottom.

**Figure E.2: The pyramid of competence**

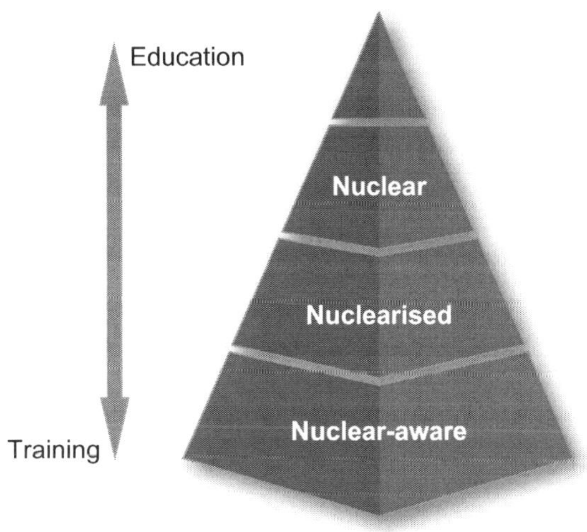


Typically, as one moves from the base to the tip of the pyramid, the acquisition of competencies shifts from training focused on a particular job, task or set of tasks, towards education, developing more in-depth underlying principles that, when properly acquired, can be applied to a less predefined set of circumstances.

Education and training, sometimes viewed as two distinct processes, are intertwined for the preparation of a competent nuclear workforce. Traditionally, vocational entrance has been associated with a stronger training component, while professional routes employ a more educative approach. Pathways are now less rigidly separated, with a necessary degree of interchange to match the development needs of employees. Industry has, in some instances, reacted to the shortage of the technical workforce by recruiting people with adequate competencies in relevant areas but without a nuclear background, which has been imparted to these new recruits through specific training. Industry has also supplemented staff with increasingly large contractor supply chains, in which there is a pressing need to establish and maintain a strong safety culture. This issue is a matter of continual review by safety authorities, as reported in the 2009 NEA Committee on the Safety of Nuclear Installations (CSNI) Technical Opinion Paper on *Improving Human and Organisational Performance*.

Nuclear professionals at the top of the pyramid are crucially important for the research, development and design leading to the safe operation of nuclear installations. This top stratum (which was the focus of the *Cause for Concern* report) is where most nuclear power plant managers can be classified. They are essential for transmitting nuclear safety culture to the entire workforce. For this category, education in nuclear engineering and/or nuclear physics, or experience in non-power nuclear applications (e.g. nuclear navies), are typically a prerequisite. This education is often provided by higher education institutions through bachelor's or master's programmes. In addition, depending on the role, training on simulators (e.g. for reactor operators) and other forms of specific on-the-job training are also required before reaching full professional competence.

Doctoral programmes are necessary to educate a number of specialists and to develop researchers in nuclear science and engineering, and are indispensable for supporting research and development in the industry and research institutions as well as for university teaching.

Since the 2000 NEA report, further concerns were subsequently uncovered with respect to an insufficient supply of operators and technicians to support existing nuclear power plants through their (extended) lifetimes. In the United States, for instance, industry workforce surveys indicate that this constitutes the greatest near-term US workforce need. With prospects of new build and as a part of the growth of nuclear industry on a global scale, even greater attention will be required for the training of the larger part of the nuclear workforce, often transient, forming the base of the pyramid.

Bearing in mind the long lead times generally required for nuclear education and training, the establishment and preservation of an adequate nuclear workforce supply calls for systematic planning decades ahead. In this respect, contradictory energy policies can have grave effects. A deteriorated global context caused by the persistent financial crisis and the negative sentiments in the wake of the Fukushima Daiichi accident heighten uncertainties and may exacerbate existing shortcomings. Indeed, shifting or deferred government decisions act as deterrent mechanisms in investment and employment, and have deleterious repercussions on the interest and engagement of younger people in the industry.

Coherent intervention by governments, industry, universities and research and development organisations thus remains vital to avert the risk of human resource shortages in some countries and to maintain the stock of skilled and competent workers. It is also necessary in order to ensure a flow of new recruits which is sustainable in the long term and adequate, in particular, to offset impending retirements.

## Ten years on – the developments

Looking at developments over the past decade, evidence from countries suggests that, in response to persisting concerns and new market conditions, stakeholders have taken actions, albeit not immediate and often driven by external forces. Challenges have been acknowledged and progress has been achieved in addressing certain issues and recommendations raised in the 2000 NEA report. However, overall, concerns remain that a process for providing a sustainable human resource supply has not been achieved in all areas or in all countries.

### *Governments*

In many countries, the educational system is shaped by governments. Hence, while actions by other stakeholders are important, without strong government participation there is limited ability to change the educational system. However, across the board, governments have, in general, done very little of a longer-term and more strategic nature.

Experience shows that active monitoring of demand and supply capacity is a fundamental step for human resource development. However, for it to bear effective and long-lasting benefits, it should be conducted on an ongoing basis, with assessments undertaken regularly and frequently for systematic planning.

In several countries, governments have commissioned workforce assessments. In some cases, the results and recommendations drawn from such surveys triggered significant government actions to address emerging gaps. National councils and bodies have been established (e.g. in France, Japan and the United Kingdom) to undertake labour market research and workforce planning, which has often proven effective for the initiation of government actions in favour of human resource development.

Some governments have provided specific support to university programmes and research, which has contributed, in a few instances, to reversing the declining trends of subscription in nuclear engineering. In many cases, fluctuating policies or lack of long-term strategy for existing programmes contribute to producing human resource development approaches and systems that are deficient, inconsistent or inadequate, if not completely absent.

**Recommendation 1**

*Governments should show a continuous and stable engagement in human resource development planning for the long-term timescales that transcend fluctuations in economic cycles. Government involvement should include regular, active monitoring of demand and supply capacity, as well as allocation of funds to support educational programmes which provide a means of developing and maintaining specialist expertise.*

### *Education*

Universities have also striven to make improvements over the last ten years, with some new and advanced nuclear courses being launched in an increasingly global context. In some cases, and notably when assisted by governmental funding and support, academic programmes have succeeded in reversing the declining trend of student recruitments experienced during the 1980s and 1990s. This is exemplified by what has occurred in the United States and in France. Healthier numbers of students have also been attracted by the prospect of new build, or high profile research topics and international projects.

Co-ordination efforts have proved to be an effective means for the promotion or preservation of nuclear education programmes. Academic institutions have achieved this, sometimes in conjunction with other parties (e.g. research centres), through the establishment of networks, the launch of international programmes, or through the amalgamation of courses, which has been vital in countries with fading nuclear programmes or with a small demand for specialists.

Noteworthy is the creation in some countries of inter-university consortia and college partnerships, allowing early interaction with young students. Some universities have engaged with technical colleges to address the increasing demand for craft and technical skills. Some courses have been specifically devised for the "nuclearisation" of non-nuclear professionals.

However, in many countries, supply has not yet reached a sustainable level taking into account future demands.

**Recommendation 2**

*Universities should intensify efforts, in collaboration with industry, to provide a greater range of courses and with greater flexibility in means of attendance by students.*

**Recommendation 3**

*Governments should support educational institutions and nuclear technology students at technical colleges to ensure there is a well-rounded workforce available for all of the nuclear careers.*

### *Research facilities*

The integration of national research facilities and academic institutes in international frameworks has generally grown. It is widely recognised that strong research programmes, increased participation in international initiatives and greater involvement of government, industry and academia in research and training can considerably improve the attraction of high-calibre students and young researchers in the field and improve their education. This collaborative approach must continue.

Co-ordination with universities and other stakeholders has been pursued by research organisations, namely through direct participation in academic curricula, the promotion and delivery of courses and seminars to a varied audience, the offer of internships, the provision of well-equipped laboratories and guidance to domestic and foreign students for their research, the awarding of prizes, grants and fellowships, and the organisation of visits.

Building on a recent activity developed by the European Union Sustainable Nuclear Energy Technology Platform, a survey was undertaken across NEA countries to measure the availability and level of use of nuclear research infrastructure for education and training. Owners or operators of facilities were requested to provide information by means of a questionnaire. This survey indicated a concern over the number and utilisation of research reactors in some countries. Thermal-hydraulic loops are less susceptible to obsolescence and hence there is much less concern over availability and ageing. However, they also appear to be largely underutilised for education and training. Full advantage should be taken of these existing facilities, including available industry research infrastructure. The following recommendations are based on the outcomes of this investigation.

#### Recommendation 4

*Access to research facilities suitable for education and training purposes should be widened and international co-ordination for such uses should be enhanced. Efforts should be made by governments to financially support existing infrastructure.*

#### Recommendation 5

*Research and academic institutions offering laboratory sessions, including computer simulations, should take new initiatives for the collection and preparation of pedagogical materials (books, software) in support of such sessions.*

Computer models and computer simulations do not replace laboratory sessions but can enhance theoretical understanding. The role of simulators in training is mandatory in some countries and is becoming increasingly widespread. Nonetheless, the general view remains that their use in training and education is still to be considered complementary to hands-on training.

#### Recommendation 6

*Research facilities should work with industry and academia to create opportunities for more effective use of research facilities so as to enhance education and training.*

The NEA report on *Nuclear Competence Building* testified to the deterioration of the financial situation of research institutes, in many countries due to cuts in public funding and to tough competition in the niche market where they sell their services and products. Although this outlook seems to have improved in a few countries, with funds being directed to research and development and the support of research infrastructures, concerns have been raised over the fact that many expensive and unique facilities were put into operation in the 1960s. Some of them have already been shut down as will a substantial number of others in the next few years.

### Recommendation 7

*Special attention should be directed to the needs of universities for access to relevant nuclear instrumentation and critical facilities, including research reactors to perform research and enhance education. Infrastructure support should be provided to maintain existing nuclear facilities, where these can be refurbished, or to replace them when they are obsolete.*

In this regard, the example of the United States is noted, where the Department of Energy supports over 20 university research reactors and has funded nuclear energy research and equipment upgrades at US colleges and universities.

## *Industry*

The engagement of industry has generally been consistent and vigorous across the board. In the past few years, in view of a prospective nuclear renaissance, major industrial players succeeded in ramping up their recruitment rates worldwide.

Sometimes industry initiatives have also led to commendable examples of collaboration with universities and other parties, such as the funding of chairs and the sponsoring of educational and research programmes, the direct involvement in the development and delivery of courses, the offer of internships and, in some cases, the opening of research infrastructure to students.

In some countries, the industry has also been engaged in the monitoring process of human resource demand and supply and has fruitfully partnered with local universities and community colleges to address emerging gaps across different levels. Of particular note is the industry participation and initiative in the establishment of multilateral education networks. The partnership between US utilities and technical colleges has created the Nuclear Uniform Curriculum Program to address the supply of technicians in the United States. Some existing networks such as the University Network of Excellence in Nuclear Engineering and the European Nuclear Education Network are considering expanding their scope to train technical personnel, which is fully supported.

### Recommendation 8

*Networks such as those developed for educational programmes should be expanded to cover technical training as well.*

Most major industrial actors have developed and maintained strong internal vocational training processes to prepare their personnel and to ensure re-staffing. In some cases, large training centres and programmes have been set up to satisfy the high and diverse recruitment needs. However, as discussed above, attrition is still acute and in some countries the industry has been unable to retain professionals and has suffered a drain of nuclear skills towards other sectors or, in an increasingly globalised context, towards other countries.

Typically, if favourable conditions are instated, careers in the nuclear sector offer the appealing prospect of highly secure and long-term employment, which represents a point of strength of the industry.

### Recommendation 9

*In order to attract and retain high-calibre young professionals and avert cross-sector and cross-boundary attrition, the industry should provide competitive remuneration, career opportunities and recognition.*

One continual challenge facing the nuclear industry is maintaining and continuously enhancing safety culture, which is difficult to measure. A further challenge comes from the fact that the few multinational suppliers are confronted with many different standards and codes, as well as the diversity produced by a global supply chain.

### *Internationalisation*

A general tendency characterising the sector has been the significant and increasing internationalisation. With a consolidated market of few global technology vendors and progressively more research and development projects developed across national borders, recent years have witnessed an increased globalisation of the civil nuclear industry and its supply chain. Nuclear power has become an international business bounded by international agreements. Greater emphasis has been placed on international collaboration for regulation, basic research and development, as well as the intricate global supply chains involving utilities, vendors and contractors in manufacturing, engineering, construction, operations, maintenance and decommissioning.

In connection with the increased internationalisation, new questions and issues have emerged, such as student and human resource mobility, quality control of education and training, greater understanding of different nuclear job profiles, and the need for a set of transferable nuclear competencies and safety awareness that support an international supply chain.

This has prompted many international initiatives. The various new programmes of international and intergovernmental bodies have given rise to means by which organisations may source or collaborate on research, education, training and knowledge management at a range of levels internationally, and instruments by which they can also draw from and contribute to labour market research on the supply and demand of human resources in nuclear energy.

Global partnerships committed to enhancing international education and leadership in the peaceful application of nuclear science and technology have been established in the last few years, such as the World Nuclear University and the European Nuclear Energy Leadership Academy. The role of the European Commission in supporting human resource development has been particularly noteworthy and has resulted in many new initiatives such as the European Nuclear Education Network, the European Fission Training Schemes, the European Human Resource Observatory in the Nuclear Energy Sector and the European Nuclear Safety and Security School.

#### Recommendation 10

*Governments should strongly encourage and support international initiatives and programmes, which foster consistent quality of the education and training being delivered in different countries and overall contribute to enhancing human resource development capacities.*

In this new context, in addition to the duties of countries with respect to existing national programmes, there is the emerging responsibility of providers and vendors to develop a competent workforce in recipient countries. Various bilateral and multilateral agreements have been established at different levels (institutional, academic and industrial) and numerous transnational education and training projects have been initiated in several countries. Yet, even with the international components emerging in the nuclear industry and increasingly in education, the responsibility for national education ultimately remains with individual governments.

Countries with strong national nuclear activities, facilities and resources have initiated programmes to "train the trainers", which complement similar programmes conceived by international organisations (notably the International Atomic Energy Agency). These are implemented in close co-operation with interested countries and specifically tailored to their needs and local education systems with the aim of forming a strong pool of indigenous human resources.

The uptake of transnational programmes as well as regional and national networks has often benefitted from improved technological means. Novel communication systems and IT instruments can be more appealing to new generations, and their dissemination has allowed the development of effective and innovative learning methods. Increasingly, web-based resources as well as distance learning are embraced as common practices both by education and research institutions as well as industry training programmes. This has helped to enlarge the pool of prospective students. Through distance learning, students can take courses even when these are not available at their own university, during a semester when they may not be taught, or, importantly, when physical or geographical obstacles would prevent their physical attendance or make it significantly more onerous. However, this raises the issue of consistency and certification.

## Job taxonomy

Recognising this emerging internationalisation of the workforce and the overarching priority to ensure safety, and drawing from the experience of a number of countries, the expert group responsible for this study researched and classified a set of job roles with significant nuclear competence that are found across the nuclear industry. This effort laid the basis for the development of a classification system for nuclear job profiles: a job taxonomy framework.

The proposed taxonomic system is of course nominal. It is neither a final nor a unique solution, but it provides a first step to assist the development of classifications.

Nuclear job specifications have been produced for the main activities associated with the construction, operation and decommissioning of commercial and research reactors, drawing up on analyses conducted by a number of companies. These may serve as an initial platform on which organisations or governments can overlay their own specific requirements.

An analysis of commonalities has led to the following findings and recommendations:

- Competence in technical and regulatory matters features consistently and prominently in nuclear job specifications across the globe. Nuclear safety culture is inextricably linked to both.
- Information, advice and guidance on training, especially concerning technical and regulatory competencies, could be improved through accreditation of training, whether provided in-house or outsourced.
- There are limited international occupational standards to guide nuclear training and workforce development,[1] although there are national standards such as those established by the Institute of Nuclear Power Operations in the United States.[2]
- Apart from the National Nuclear Accreditation Board in the United States and the National Skills Academy in the United Kingdom, there are no other independent national bodies for the accreditation of nuclear training.
- Taxonomy as a tool in workforce development can aid workforce planning in elaborating scenarios for the supply and demand of skills, in developing training standards, and as a structure for competence assurance management systems such as nuclear passport schemes.
- Both governments and employers can benefit from access to high-quality labour market intelligence and training standards. This can inform, for example, targeted policy interventions such as directives on training or prioritisation of resources for higher education and research.
- Dissemination of international guidelines for training and competence assurance would assist employers in choosing or designing appropriate workforce development programmes.

### Recommendation 11

Drawing from the experience of the National Nuclear Accreditation Board in the United States, it is recommended that:

*Consideration should be given to carrying over to training the accreditation and certification culture that is well established in education, and to establishing independent accreditation and certification of training provision and employer schemes.*

1. It is noted that at a European level there is a strong drive to structuring training and career development across the EU and to establishing European high-quality "reference standards" with the ultimate objective of creating a European competence passport.
2. It is worth noting that the work done by the Institute of Nuclear Power Operations (INPO) for operators is distributed internationally by the World Association of Nuclear Operators (WANO).

Safety culture permeates nuclear job specifications. In this regard, the proposed taxonomy brings into prominence not only the competence assurance considerations of the previous section, but also the technical and regulatory competencies, both of which relate to safety.

### Recommendation 12

There appears to be international consensus on the fundamental components of basic nuclear training covering fundamental technical and regulatory matters to support the production of an outline programme in "basic nuclear awareness" that could have value for the international community. It is therefore recommended that:

*Consideration should be given to the provision of an outline for training in "basic nuclear awareness" with content adequate to cover both the range of nuclear sectors and the range of occupational levels.*

## Reference

Li, N., C. Dale, K. Kern and S. Scott (2009), "Los Alamos Nuclear Enterprise Resource and Infrastructure Model (LA-NERIM)", Los Alamos National Laboratory, Proc. International Congress on Advances in Nuclear Power Plants 2009 (ICAPP 2009), 10-14 May 2009, Shinjuku, Tokyo, Japan.

# *Chapter 1*
# A decade of change

## 1.1 Background

In 2000, the Nuclear Energy Agency published *Nuclear Education and Training: Cause for Concern?* (NEA, 2000), which, for the first time, drew attention to the likelihood of insufficient human resources being available to support current operations, foreseeable developments and the decommissioning of shut-down nuclear facilities. A number of measures were proposed in the report to encourage urgent intervention by key stakeholders. Governments were identified as needing to set long-term strategic energy plans, including consideration of skilled workforce demand; universities were tasked with pursuing the development of attractive educational programmes; and industry was directed towards the support of effective training programmes.

Progress against the recommendations was assessed in 2004 in a follow-up report, *Nuclear Competence Building* (NEA, 2004). A number of outstanding problems were highlighted particularly connected with the time required to accumulate sufficient skills and knowledge to achieve competence, a situation made worse by a loss of existing experience, a contraction in research and training facilities, and reduced university funding. Although awareness of the overall future skills deficit had occurred, it was concluded that the response was geographically variable, and it was noted that there had been no universal breakthrough in addressing the demographic downturn. Some additional recommendations were added and earlier ones reiterated. Areas to be addressed included: international collaboration across government, industry and academia; regular workforce surveys; and increased support for research and development (R&D).

In 2007, the NEA Steering Committee for Nuclear Energy unanimously adopted a statement on the need for qualified human resources in the nuclear field, and noted the explicit role for government in ensuring its availability (NEA, 2007). The three central issues were:

- maintaining skills over the lifetime of existing nuclear power plants (NPPs) including decommissioning, against the backdrop, in some countries, of licence extensions;
- developing and retaining skilled workers in other nuclear facilities related to the nuclear fuel cycle, such as waste management and reprocessing;
- dealing with the ageing workforce.

In the intervening period the political and technological landscape has changed considerably with an increased global opportunity for civil nuclear power and with a demand for an expanding skilled nuclear workforce. Some initiatives have been successfully launched to halt the decline of the numbers of highly educated and trained workforce, although concerns remain that a long-term approach is still lacking in many countries, while the workforce as a whole is still ageing.

Furthermore, over the last ten years, nuclear education and training has evolved against a more nuanced understanding of how nuclear skills need to be addressed.

Against this backdrop the present study was initiated under the auspices of the NEA Committee for Technical and Economic Studies on Nuclear Energy Development and the Fuel Cycle. In late 2009 an ad hoc expert group was established to develop the work, with consultant support; the detailed list of experts is provided in Appendix 6.

Whilst a systematic quantitative assessment was envisaged in the original scope of the study, this was not conducted, as other parallel initiatives were announced in the course of the work [notably the global survey proposed by International Atomic Energy Agency (IAEA) at the International Conference on Human Resource Development – Abu Dhabi 14-18 March 2010].[1] Complementary but equally fundamental aspects of the resourcing of the nuclear industry have therefore been addressed, capitalising on the group's expertise.

This study assesses the current state of education and training for the development of nuclear skills development, the remaining gaps, and the actions that are now required to address corresponding needs across NEA member countries. Programmes and instruments for human resource development (HRD) have been covered in a threefold fashion: 1) by looking at the provision of the specialist nuclear education for nuclear professionals through the appraisal of initiatives that have been undertaken over the last ten years by the various actors in the international scene; 2) through a parallel survey on the use of research facilities for education and training; and 3) through the development of a job taxonomy consisting in mapping-out and typifying various nuclear job profiles.

## 1.2 The evolving environment

Nuclear power has played an important role in addressing global issues related to energy demand, climate change mitigation and security of supply. The increasing world demand for energy has strengthened the position of nuclear power, giving it a strategic importance within nation states, and globally as the international community responds to population growth and a sharply rising demand for low-carbon sources of electricity as a way to mitigate climate change.

### *1.2.1 The strategic role of nuclear electricity generation*

This section briefly discusses the principal drivers that will support the continued need for nuclear power and the general context in which this is developed and therefore why nuclear education and training will remain a crucial and pressing need for the industry into the foreseeable future.

*Economic growth and energy demand*

Global economic growth and development rely on electricity as a high value, versatile energy carrier. Although short-term total energy demand tends to track the rise and fall of the prevailing economic environment, the longer-term outlook remains upwards, with electricity showing the most aggressive increase of any final-form energy. Indeed, a correspondence can be demonstrated between electricity use and the UN Human Development Index, implying that such an increase is intrinsically linked to economic and social progress (at least up to a certain level of electricity consumption). The scale of this trend is such that by 2050, global electricity production could increase to about 2.5 times its current level (IEA, 2010), if the existing expansion in population and attendant economic activity is maintained.

Although the largest rate of growth is, and is expected to remain, in developing countries, the industrialised world is itself a growing consumer. Within the OECD group, electricity generation increased by 2.9% per year between 1971 and 2007, similar to the GDP growth rate (NEA, 2008). This poses a particular challenge for the long-term provision of sufficient electricity in a way which is secure and of limited environmental impact.

*Environmental drivers*

A number of international reports address climate change and the relationship to the amounts of atmospheric $CO_2$ and other "greenhouse" gases (e.g. IPCC, 2007 and 2008). Although some controversies have arisen, a scientific consensus is shared by the governments that are party to the

1. www.iaea.org/inisnkm/nkm/pages/2010/conference_UAE_March_2010.htm.

United Nations Framework Convention on Climate Change (UNFCCC).[2] The International Panel on Climate Change (IPCC) reports that electricity production is responsible for 27% of anthropomorphic greenhouse gas production. To achieve a major decarbonisation of electricity generation, nuclear could play a role, since it produces virtually no greenhouse gas emissions during operation.

### *Energy security*

Many countries are attracted to nuclear power because it can supply reliable, affordable, safe base load electric power with virtually no gas emissions of greenhouse gases. It avoids the dependency on oil, coal and gas, whose prices have shown wide fluctuation and which are sourced (in the case of much of the oil and gas) from countries subject to political instability. On the other hand, geological deposits of uranium are widely distributed through largely politically stable regions. In addition, estimates of the reserves of uranium imply sufficient fissile material for many decades to come. The OECD/NEA and the IAEA report *Uranium 2009: Resources, Production and Demand* identified conventional uranium resources at 6.3 MtU (NEA, 2010). According to this report the uranium resources are expected to be sufficient for at least another 100 years of supply (at 2008 reactor requirement levels) and production is expected to be more than adequate to meet the demand in the near term, even for high growth scenarios, provided that existing and committed plans of capacity expansion are achieved in a timely manner. Moreover, continued advancements in nuclear fuel utilisation and the deployment of advanced (breeder) reactors would also further improve long-term viability.

### *Economics*

The cost of generating electricity varies between technologies, not only in the overall price but in the contributions of fixed capital and variable costs, sensitivity to fuel prices, the cost profile over the lifetime of the power plant and whether the source provides baseload, dispatchable or intermittent generation. Despite these complicating factors, it is possible to take account of different characteristics to undertake meaningful comparisons. The International Energy Agency (IEA) and the NEA publish regular assessments based on the notion of levelised costs of electricity (LCOE), that is, the breakeven point for investment for the lifetime of the plant. In 2010, the report *Projected Costs of Generating Electricity* (IEA/NEA, 2010), indicated that nuclear power is the most competitive option at a discount rate of 5% and assuming a carbon price of USD 30 per tonne of $CO_2$ emitted. This was true for all regions. At a 10% discount rate, the competitiveness of nuclear fell behind gas in Europe but remained the most competitive in Asia.

The largest contribution to the cost of nuclear generated electricity is from capital costs during construction. These are determined by a variety of elements, mostly related to the plant design and the financing of lengthy times of construction. Advanced designs offer the prospect of more efficient and safer systems, using fewer components and lower costs. However most are still in a first-of-a-kind stage and so it has not yet been demonstrated if capital costs can be significantly reduced. Actions are being undertaken to minimise lead times, for instance by optimising the planning and licence approval processes. The greatest investment return is obtained where multi-reactor, large capacity plants can be built efficiently and designed to operate for 40 years and beyond. Reductions in costs can be achieved through longer lifetimes, improved capacity factors and technological advancements, including the introduction of simplified, standardised, and to an extent modularised designs. These would make nuclear energy more attractive, both in terms of the LCOE as well as in terms of reduction of investor risks.

Operational lifetimes are now routinely expected to reach and exceed 60 years. Lifetime extensions, based on comprehensive safety reviews, have been widely implemented. With most components being replaceable, lifetimes of 50 to 60 years are now feasible through the substitution of ageing equipment and upgrade of systems to enhance safety and increase efficiency.

2. www.unfccc.int.

In 2000, at the time of the publication of *Cause for Concern*, the trajectory of the nuclear industry was still undergoing restraints generated by safety concerns and cheap fossil fuels in the 1990s, and the contribution nuclear could make to address environmental concerns was not fully recognised. A decade later, the political and public attitude to nuclear generation had changed markedly. In brief, and at the time of writing, highlights of statistics in the nuclear sector are (IAEA, 2012 and 2012a):

- 436 power reactors operational worldwide;
- 139 power reactors have been shut down;
- 63 power reactors under construction;
- 244 research reactors worldwide (232 operational and 12 temporarily in shutdown), usually housed by research institutes (including universities);
- 202 research or prototype reactors in decommissioning;

Significantly, the largest number of new reactors under construction has been obtained in these last years (65 new reactors were under construction in 2011), since 1992 (IAEA, 2011). Assessments made by the NEA and IEA (among others) before the Fukushima Daiichi accident, showed global nuclear capacity reaching 475-500 GWe by 2020; up to 13 GWe per year. The annual rate of construction starts is not however high by historical measures. In the year 2010 there were 16 new nuclear construction starts, compared with an average of over 25 per year throughout the 1970s (IAEA, 2010). Lifetime extension has contributed substantially to maintaining the capacity in various countries. National policies towards nuclear development vary from government to government, depending on political priorities, local resources and the strategic weight assigned to the technology by each country. A number of states have set nuclear generation targets, while others are content to allow market demand signals to determine how many reactors, and of which type, are built. In the aftermath of the Fukushima Daiichi accident some countries have decided to forgo new nuclear development and have set a timetable to close their existing plants over the next several years (notably Germany and Switzerland). However, other countries have reaffirmed their nuclear plans to supply needed electricity while meeting environmental commitments.

Given a lead time of up to a decade for new build, the nuclear infrastructure for 2020 is already largely planned. Major areas of expansion are centred on China, India and Russia, but established networks in Canada, the Czech Republic, Korea, Lithuania, Romania, South Africa, the United Kingdom and the United States are also the subject of planned growth. Some states with no existing capacity are considering installation, including Poland, Turkey and the UAE (NEA, 2010a).

### 1.2.2 Specific aspects of nuclear power

Some of the distinctive features and challenges which characterise nuclear energy and make education and training in this sector very different from other forms of industrial training are discussed in this section.

In particular, nuclear power is subject to comprehensive regulatory oversight and high-levels of design standards, construction and operation. Nuclear requires therefore a cohort of regulators, operators, managers and support personnel technically well qualified and with a very strong safety awareness and a wide range of skills and competencies.

#### *Safety*

Radiation control, safety in operations and effective regulation are fundamental aspects of nuclear power. Safety remains the pre-eminent concern throughout the lifetime of nuclear facilities. For instance, for the construction of new nuclear power plants, governments are required to operate a rigorous assessment procedure in granting broad consent, examining not only the safety of the technology but also the appropriateness, environmental impacts and security of the proposed location and associated supply routes.

 NUCLEAR EDUCATION AND TRAINING: FROM CONCERN TO CAPABILITY, ISBN 978-92-64-17637-9, © OECD 2012

Although probabilistic safety assessment shows the risk of severe accidents in the nuclear power sector to compare favourably with other energy chains, public confidence is very sensitive to specific nuclear incidents and severe accidents than to such type of events within other energy chains. Accidents at Three Mile Island in 1979 and Chernobyl in 1986 precipitated a collapse in public support for the industry in many countries, support that has been increasing over the last decade. Following the accident at Fukushima Daiichi public opinion has been strongly affected and the reactions of countries have varied depending on their individual circumstances. Most countries are expected to proceed with their plans for new nuclear plants, albeit at a slower pace following the accident.

Safety, security and radiation protection imply the existence of a comprehensive system of quality assurance and quality controls. For new build, although most large scale infrastructure projects are subject to considerable review, the unique status of nuclear power has in many countries added time and skill overheads. These are very specific to the nuclear sector and present in all its activities, justifying specific training. In addition, a small but critical cohort of highly skilled regulators is required to provide an objective, informed and independent verification of safety.

*Decommissioning and waste disposal*

Waste disposal from operations and end of service decommissioning are significant tasks, which must be considered as part of the complete life cycle of nuclear facilities. In some countries, such as the United Kingdom, in recent years, the decommissioning sector has formed the largest part of the civil nuclear workforce. Crucially many of the skills and behaviours associated with the decommissioning process also apply to operations when combined with appropriate re-skilling. Hence, it is expected that in such countries, if necessary, the staff transitioning from decommissioning can represent a ready stream of nuclear aware personnel for new build.

Many surveys have shown that the long-term management of spent fuel and other high-level waste remains central to public support for nuclear expansion. Indeed the implementation of deep geological disposal remains a key challenge and priority for the industry and for governments. Important advancements in this direction have been achieved in several cases (notably in Finland and Sweden) and several countries operate underground research laboratories with a view to developing geological disposal protocols and establishing long-term performance. A cadre of researchers with R&D skills in fields including hydrology, geology and actinide chemistry needs to be maintained to develop repositories which perform well and maintain public confidence.

### *1.2.3 The continuing need for human resource*

The distinctive characteristics of nuclear energy and its fuel cycle provide special requirements for education and training (E&T). In all countries with a nuclear programme, even before new build is taken into account and regardless of national policies, there exists a substantial nuclear estate to be safely operated, maintained. Intricate global supply chains involving utilities, vendors and contractors in manufacturing, engineering, construction, operations, maintenance and decommissioning attend activities across the lifecycle of the nuclear reactor, bringing extensive direct employment. An essential complement for the implementation and safe operations of all nuclear facilities and the associated research and development is a knowledgeable and skilled workforce.

Highly skilled workforces involved are substantial and constitute a significant element of the costs of building and operating nuclear power plants. It may be surprising, therefore, that there are no robust estimates of the global workforce. The situation is reflected by the example of the international publication *Nuclear Energy Outlook* (NEA, 2008) which devotes a single page out of a total of over 450 to "Quantifying Workforce Needs".

In recognition of the gap in manpower data, the IAEA has recently launched a global Nuclear Power Human Resource Survey,[3] intending to cover every NPP operator across the world and to collect comprehensive information that captures all of the different types of personnel that are currently applied to support operating nuclear power programmes. At a European level, the newly established European Human Resource Observatory Nuclear will produce and regularly update a quality-assured database on the supply and demand of human resources. In the United States the Nuclear Energy Institute performs surveys of utility workforce needs.

Estimates of workforce needs published by some individual nations (e.g. France, the United Kingdom and the United States) indicate future manpower demand in the tens-to-hundreds of thousands of skilled workers. In this respect the nuclear industry faces the dual challenge of an ageing workforce and a decline in the pool of people with recent construction experience, limitations that are exacerbated by the long lead times for nuclear training. Without coherent interventions by industry, governments and universities, severe workforce shortages in the arena of commercial nuclear plants may still emerge, mainly attributable to more than two decades of stasis in demand for new civilian plants and the increasing numbers of retirees.

A recent study by the Los Alamos Nuclear Enterprise Resource and Infrastructure simulated human resource development needs for a number of scenarios in the Russian Federation and the United States (Li *et al.*, 2009). Figure 1.1 shows the magnitude of the prospective demand for operations personnel (i.e. operating staff retained for plant operations following the construction phase) for the United States case where additional plants are built to retain market share. Starting from the 56 000 United States workforce (as of 2006) the graph shows separately staff needs to replace retiring personnel and to cater for additional capacity, indicating a demand, by 2030, of approximately 19 000 new positions and a total of 63 000 new hires (19 000 + 44 000 to replace retiring employees). The main outcome from this analysis is that there will be a large need for training and education of new employees.[4]

**Figure 1.1: Estimates of the operating personnel needed for retaining market share in nuclear power in the United States**

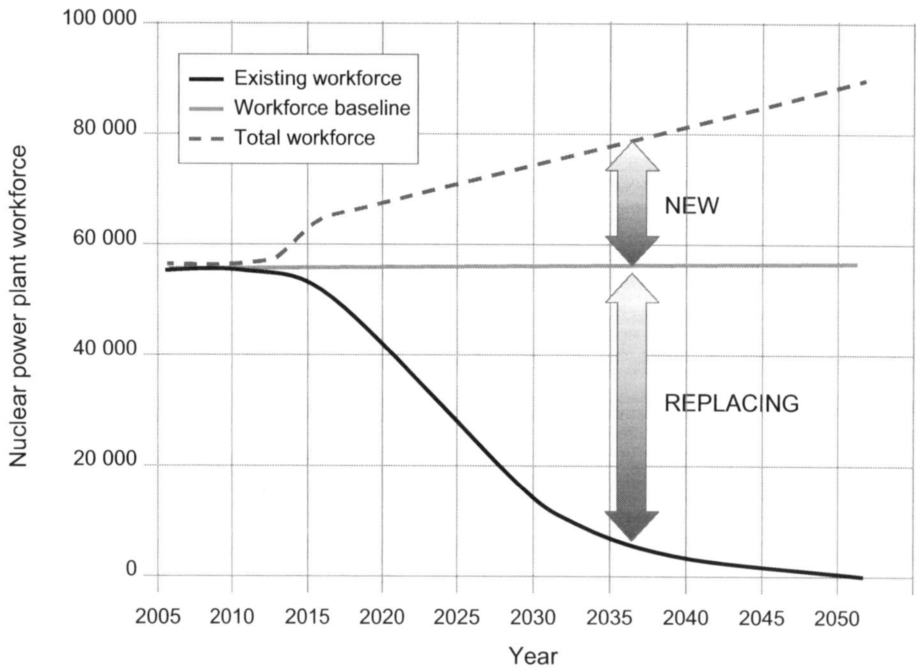


Source: Li *et al.* (2009).

3. http://iaeaglobalworkforce.org/survey/workforcesurvey.asp.

4. Similarly, in France, the figures derived from a 2008 study (OPIIEC, 2008) report that about 13 000 graduates (master level) and about 10 000 technicians will be needed in the next ten years.


NUCLEAR EDUCATION AND TRAINING: FROM CONCERN TO CAPABILITY, ISBN 978-92-64-17637-9, © OECD 2012

Other noted estimates are:

- An analysis conducted in 2009 by the US National Commission on Energy Policy, showing that the development and construction phases of a nuclear power plant project requires 14 360 (4 785 salaried and 9 575 hourly) man-years per GW installed, including a broad spread of profiles: from the predominant cohort of skilled crafts, to professionals, project managers, construction supervisors, etc.
- An independent study conducted in 2011 by Price-Waterhouse-Coopers (PWC, 2011), on average 2 700 direct jobs are needed during the design and construction phase of a European pressurised reactor in France (~ 8 350 in total, including indirect jobs). To support its operation and dismantling, the direct jobs needed are of the order of 500 (~ 1 650 in total, including indirect jobs).
- The UK Cogent report *Next Generation Skills for New Build Nuclear* of the "Renaissance Nuclear Skills Series". In this report it is assumed that, for a single twin-unit reactor, employment peaks close to 2 500 full-time equivalents (which corresponds to a full year of employment on normal working hours and leave). The study estimates that, for an indicative 16 GWe new build scenario (6 twin-unit stations) in the United Kingdom, up to 140 000 person years will be needed, with a peak (excluding manufacturing) in the total integrated workforce of 14 000.

Estimates of peak staffing during construction are reported to range from ~ 2 000 to 6 000 personnel (depending on the type of reactor, its capacity, whether it is a single or twin-unit, etc.) (IAEA, 2011*a*; Li *et al.*, 2009; Cogent, 2010).

Although individual estimates vary somewhat, depending on the national context, the different types of reactors considered and the construction cycles (for new build), it is clear that strains in resourcing the nuclear industry are still high.

In addition to this largest section of the nuclear workforce needed for NPP construction, operation and decommissioning, a well resourced R&D activity is also crucially important for current and future developments. At one extreme, research can address specific site issues and be a source of expert opinion in determining national policy directions. At the other, it reveals and matures new technologies, to support, *inter alia,* long-term waste disposal, novel reactor technologies and fuel cycles. But equally important is the mediating role research plays in informing teaching, attracting students, and stimulating international collaborations and alliances. Research sponsored by government will generally support longer-term or more fundamental projects, whereas commercial organisations promote work likely to provide benefit in the near-term.

In general, the demand for nuclear skills set against a generally ageing workforce, implies that significant intervention will be required to maintain the stock of a skilled and competent workforce, and the flow of new recruits for long-term sustainability. Policy decisions need to be made now to ensure that adequate nuclear education and training infrastructure is available in the decades ahead. Delays and changes in policies will have detrimental effects on sustaining an adequate workforce supply.

From its beginning in the twenty-first century to the present, much of the nuclear industry has shifted from the public to the private sector as the technology has matured from its post-war origins in national research and development programmes. The industry has thus become, in the course of half a century, an international business bounded by international agreements. As a result, the investments of national governments have overall shifted towards greater emphasis on international collaboration for basic research and development, on regulation, and less on direct procurement. Research and development of reactor technology are increasingly taking place across international borders. Concurrently the civil nuclear deployment and its associated supply chain have undergone internationalisation. As a result, the need has emerged for a more globalised nuclear workforce.

## 1.3 A key resource – a competent workforce

The nuclear industry is characterised by a requirement for high overall skill levels and a high degree of safety. Safety is a pre-eminent concern in the nuclear industry overwhelmingly for its own sake, but also its sensitivity in term of public perception and, formally because of national and regional regulations and international agreements, such as the Convention on Nuclear Safety.[5] The importance of training and education in maintaining safety cannot be understated (IAEA).[6] For all of these reasons, safe behaviours are regarded as critical skills that sit in parallel with the specific technical competencies for the job. Managers and leaders have a key role to model appropriate behaviours and to support nuclear education and training in order to generate and maintain a robust safety culture.

It is useful to recognise that there exist various degrees of "nuclearisation" within the industry; that is, the extent to which specific nuclear skills and safety culture training augment other engineering or management skills. Throughout the workforce, general nuclear awareness is a prerequisite, with more specialised nuclear expertise being required by fewer personnel, depending on the specific job requirements. The emphasis, then, is in adding skills in depth, as appropriate, to the job role and tasks contained within.

A threefold categorisation of the competencies necessary to run a nuclear power station can be drawn, which includes:

- "nuclear" people with a specialised formal education in nuclear subjects (e.g. nuclear engineering, radiochemistry, radiation protection, etc.);
- "nuclearised" people with formal education and training in a relevant (non-nuclear) area (e.g. mechanical, electrical, civil engineering, systems) but who need to acquire knowledge of the nuclear environment in which they have to apply their competencies;
- "nuclear aware" people requiring nuclear awareness to work in the industry (e.g. electricians, mechanics, and other crafts and support personnel).

This can be visualised in terms of the pyramid of competence in Figure 1.2. Generally there will be a larger number of employees from top to bottom.

**Figure 1.2: The pyramid of competence**

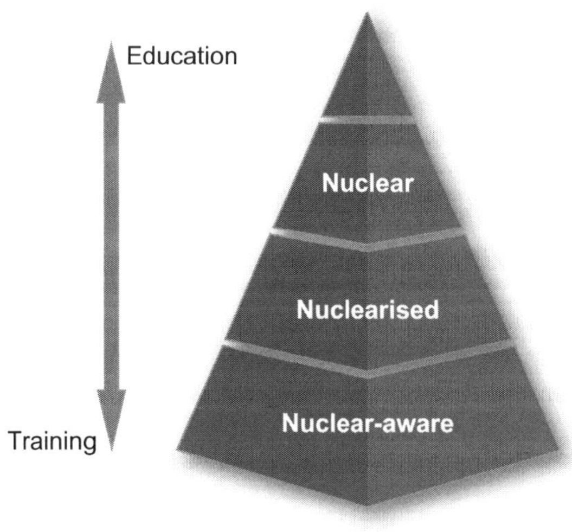


5. www.iaea.org/Publications/Documents/Infcircs/Others/inf449.shtml.
6. Advisory Group Meeting on Education and Training in Nuclear Safety, IAEA, Vienna, 2001.


NUCLEAR EDUCATION AND TRAINING: FROM CONCERN TO CAPABILITY, ISBN 978-92-64-17637-9, © OECD 2012

Typically, with increasing height above the base, the acquisition route of competencies shifts from training focused on a particular job, task or set of tasks, towards education, developing more in-depth underlying principles that, when properly acquired, can be applied to a less predefined set of circumstances.

Traditionally, vocational entrance has been associated with a stronger training component, while professional routes employ a more educative approach:

- education refers to the in-depth acquisition of knowledge in the discipline; it includes theoretical courses (e.g. mathematics and physics), laboratory sessions, practical applications, and may include theses and internships;
- training refers to the acquisition of skills, including all necessary knowledge (i.e. focused education) to achieve a competence to work in a particular specific environment.

Although sometimes held as two distinct processes, education and training are often intertwined for the preparation of a competent nuclear workforce. Progressively pathways have become less rigidly separated, with a degree of interchange to match the development needs of employees. Industry has, for instance, reacted to the shortage of technical workforce by also recruiting people with adequate competencies in relevant areas but without a nuclear background, which gets imparted through specific training. Industry has also supplemented staff with increasingly large contractor supply chains, for whom there is a pressing need to establish and maintain a strong safety culture. This issue is a matter of concern for safety authorities, as reported in the last NEA/CSNI Technical Opinion Paper on Improving Human and Organisational Performance (NEA, 2009).

Nuclear professionals at the top of the pyramid are crucially important for the operation of nuclear installations, not least for their function of transmitting nuclear safety culture to the entire workforce (this top stratum was the focus of the *Cause for Concern* report). For this category, education in nuclear engineering and/or nuclear physics, or experience in non-commercial nuclear applications (e.g. nuclear navies and R&D), are typically a prerequisite. This education is often provided by higher education institutions through bachelor's or master's programmes.

Depending on the specific role, training on simulators (e.g. for reactor operators) and specific on-the-job accreditation (e.g. technicians) is also required before reaching full professional competence.

Doctoral programmes are necessary to educate a number of specialists and to develop researchers in nuclear science and engineering and are indispensable for supporting R&D in the industry and research institutions and for university teaching.

Interconnections between different aspects of the process are represented in Figure 1.3, which reflects the important interactions among industry, universities and government in producing a competent workforce with the right mixture of knowledge and skills. The IAEA publication *Status and Trends in Nuclear Education*, from which the figure is derived, points out that co-operation is critical in both creating and maintaining education and training programmes and in attracting young people towards nuclear engineering (IAEA, 2010a). Equally importantly, it allows the skills demand to tune educational programmes to provide a better match with industrial needs. With the generic underpinning established, industry is then able to focus on the specific additions required in the work place.

In practical terms, industrial and academic co-operation may take a number of forms involving the exchange of students and staff, internship programmes, joint R&D projects which may also be conducted at research centres. The significant point is that it is the efficient delivery of the two learning strands, education and training, which is at the heart of a steady flow of competent workers.

**Figure 1.3: Competence pathways**

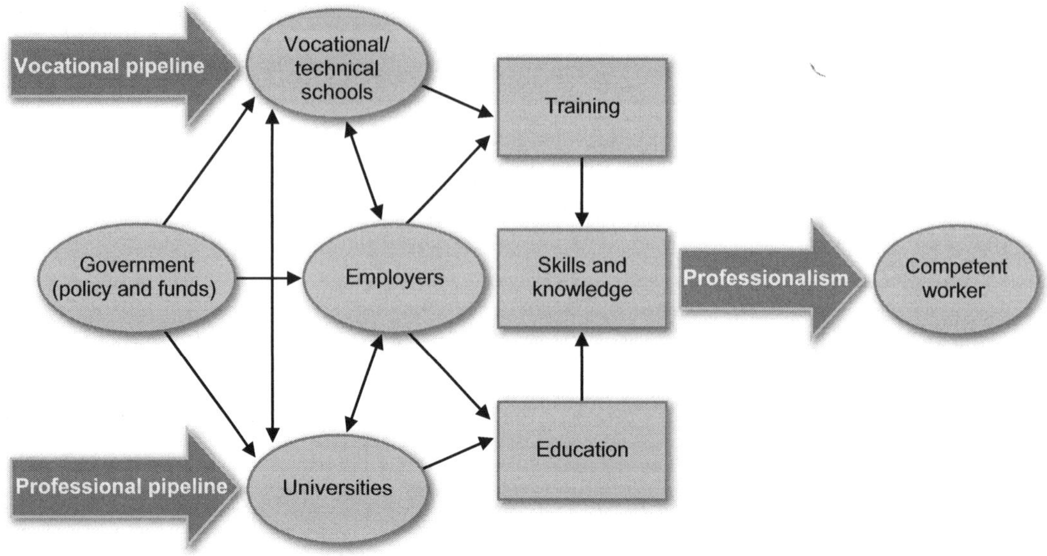


Assessment of the quality of nuclear education is achieved under the framework of the normal quality assessment of higher education institutions, leading to their validation. Accreditation is common practice in education, in the United States for example it is conducted by Accreditation Board for Engineering and Technology (ABET).[7] However, in general, the equivalent process with regard to training is less clear. It is noted that the European Commission has recently established and is promoting the European Credit system for Vocational Education and Training (ECVET). In some instances requirements for the validation of nuclear training programmes are very stringent: such is the case for the training of operators and several other categories of workers in the United States where accreditation of training is carried out by the independent National Nuclear Accreditation Board and sanctioned by the Nuclear Regulatory Commission (US NRC). However, in some countries such requirements are less clear, with the utility holding the responsibility for ensuring and demonstrating to the regulator that appropriate training processes are in place.

The focal point of the 2000 NEA report was the top of the pyramid. Further concerns were subsequently uncovered with respect to the dearth of operators and technicians needed to support existing nuclear plants through their (extended) lifetimes. With prospects of new build and as a part of the growth of a global nuclear industry, even greater attention will be required for nuclear workforce training. Most of the new jobs will be at the base of the pyramid for technicians and support staff not only for the new plants but also for the growing international supply chain. Industry workforce surveys indicate that in some countries there is a growing and persistent need for new technicians to enter the industry; in the United States, for instance, this constitutes the greatest near-term workforce need.

Furthermore, in several countries, human mobility and skills transfer have arisen as central issues.

The nuclear industry as a whole encapsulates a wide range of job and skill levels required, with descriptors that have, historically, varied from one employer to another. Codifying the total skill

7. ABET (www.abet.org) is a non-profit, non-governmental organisation that accredits college and university programmes in the disciplines of applied science, computing, engineering, and engineering technology. ABET accredits over 3 100 programmes at more than 660 colleges and universities in 23 countries. It provides specialised, programmatic accreditation that evaluates an individual programme of study, rather than evaluating an institution as a whole.

demand is essential if a responsive global industry is to develop, with the resources and flexibility to meet the world demand.

Chapter 2 of this study addresses the progress in education and training in establishing the capacity for skill development since the publication of *Cause for Concern*. Instruments already available, underway or planned are considered, with special emphasis on the preparation of professionals at the top of the pyramid. Among such instruments, the current and future uses of nuclear research facilities for E&T purposes are assessed on the basis on data gathered through quantitative surveys.

Chapter 3 provides an outline of a job classification system, or taxonomy to aid the development of skilled capacity, across the nuclear workforce, in a way which is robust, measured and consistent.

Conclusions and recommendations are presented in Chapter 4.

## References

Burgherr, P., S. Hirschberg, A. Hunt and R. A. Ortiz (2004), *Severe Accidents in the Energy Sector: Final Report to the European Commission of the EU 5th Framework Programme "New Element for the Assessment of External Costs from Energy Technologies"*, DG Research, Technological Development and Demonstration (RTD), Brussels, Belgium.

Cogent (2010), *Next Generation Skills for New Build Nuclear*, "Renaissance Nuclear Skills Series", Cogent Sector Skills Council, Warrington, United Kingdom. Available at www.cogent-scc.com/research/nuclearresearch.php.

IAEA (2010), *Nuclear Technology Review 2010*, IAEA, Vienna.

IAEA (2010a), *Status and Trends in Nuclear Education*, IAEA, Vienna. Available at www.pub.iaea.org/MTCD/publications/PDF/P1475_web.pdf.

IAEA (2011), *Power Reactor Information System*, IAEA, Vienna, Austria. Available at www.iaea.org/programmes/a2/.

IAEA (2011a), *Workforce Planning for New Nuclear Power Programmes*, IAEA, Vienna, Austria. Available at www-pub.iaea.org/books/IAEABooks/8488/Workforce-Planning-for-New-Nuclear-Power-Programmes.

IAEA (2012), *Power Reactor Information System*, IAEA, Vienna, Austria. Available at www.iaea.org/programmes/a2/.

IAEA (2012a), *IAEA Research Reactor Database (RRDB)*, IAEA, Vienna, Austria. Available at http://nucleus.iaea.org/RRDB/RR/ReactorSearch.aspx?filter=0.

IEA (2010), *Energy Technology Perspectives 2010, Scenarios & Strategies to 2050*, International Energy Agency, OECD, Paris, France.

IEA/NEA (2010), *Projected Costs of Generating Electricity*, 2010 Edition, International Energy Agency and Nuclear Energy Agency, OECD, Paris, France.

IPCC (2007), *Climate Change 2007: Mitigation*. Contribution of Working Group III to the Fourth Assessment Report of the Intergovernmental Panel on Climate Change, Summary for Policy Makers, Cambridge University Press, Cambridge, United Kingdom and New York, NY, United States.

IPCC (2008), *Climate Change 2007: Synthesis Report*, Contribution of Working Groups I, II and III to the Fourth Assessment Report of the Intergovernmental Panel on Climate Change, IPCC, Geneva, Switzerland.

Li, N., C. Dale, K. Kern and S. Scott (2009), "Los Alamos Nuclear Enterprise Resource and Infrastructure Model (LA-NERIM)", Los Alamos National Laboratory, Proc. International Congress on Advances in Nuclear Power Plants 2009 (ICAPP 2009), 10-14 May 2009, Shinjuku, Tokyo, Japan.

NEA (2000), *Nuclear Education and Training: Cause for Concern?*, OECD, Paris, France.

NEA (2004), *Nuclear Competence Building*, OECD, Paris, France

NEA (2007), *Proposed Statement by the NEA Steering Committee for Nuclear Energy regarding a Government Role in Ensuring Qualified Human Resources in the Nuclear Field*, NEA/NE(2007)9, September 2007, OECD, Paris, France.

NEA (2008), *Nuclear Energy Outlook 2008*, OECD, Paris, France.

NEA (2009), *CSNI Technical Opinion Papers No. 11 Better Nuclear Plant Maintenance: Improving Human and Organisational Performance*, OECD Nuclear Energy Agency and International Energy Agency, Paris, France.

NEA (2010), *Uranium 2009: Resources, Production and Demand*, A Joint Report by the OECD Nuclear Energy Agency and the International Atomic Energy Agency, OECD, Paris, France.

NEA (2010a), *Technology Roadmap, Nuclear Energy*, OECD Nuclear Energy Agency and International Energy Agency, Paris, France.

NEI (2009), *NEI 2009 Pipeline Survey Results*, Nuclear Energy Institute, Washington, United States.

OPIIEC (2008), Étude sur l'évolution des métiers de l'ingénierie nucléaire (Synthèse), Étude de l'OPIIEC par l'IREP, avril 2008. http://syntec.ajax.emencia.net/fr/publications/etudessurlingenierie/guidesetetudes/etudes_sectorielles/image/synthese_principaux_resultats_opiiec_nucleaire.pdf

PWC (2011), *The Socio-economic Impact of the Nuclear Power Industry in France*, Price-Waterhouse-Coopers.

*Chapter 2*

# Review of nuclear education and associated facilities

## 2.1 Introduction

Several years on since *Cause for Concern* (NEA, 2000), issues around human resource development in the nuclear industry still persist, with different issues prevailing in different countries, depending on the specifics of national nuclear programmes.

HRD is still very high in the international agenda, as it transpired in the statement (NEA, 2007) unanimously adopted in 2007 by the OECD/NEA Steering Committee. Even in later years, it has been at the heart of international reviews (IAEA, 2011; EC, 2009; Khan *et al.*, 2008) and high profile events (among the most recent, IAEA, 2010 and NESTet, 2011) and it will be the topic of the policy debate to be held by the OECD/NEA Steering Committee in 2012.

Over this past decade, in response to the persisting concerns and new market conditions, initiatives in nuclear education and training have been initiated and are still developing.

Section 2.2 of this chapter addresses the progress and challenges in establishing the education and training capacity for nuclear skill development since the publication of *Cause for Concern*. Instruments already available, underway or planned are considered, with special emphasis on the preparation of professionals. Among such instruments, the current and future uses of nuclear research facilities for E&T purposes are assessed in Section 2.3 on the basis of data gathered through quantitative surveys. Findings are reported at the end of each subsection, whereas the recommendations derived are summarised in Chapter 4.

## 2.2 Education and training – progress over the last decade

This section analyses actions undertaken by the various stakeholders: governments, universities, industries and research institutes, in NEA member countries represented within the group. Relevant changes and initiatives are appraised in relation to the individual recommendations raised in NEA, 2000 (and listed in Appendix 1). Some examples obtained, by and large through country case studies provided by delegates of the ad hoc expert group have been selected for a more in-depth discussion; others are briefly described in apposite boxes.[1] Individual country case studies are provided in full in Appendix 2.

### *2.2.1 Government initiatives*

> *Recommendation 2.A* (NEA, 2000): Governments should engage in strategic energy planning, including consideration of education, manpower and infrastructure.
>
> *Recommendation 2.B* (NEA, 2000): Governments should contribute to, if not take responsibility for, integrated planning to ensure that human resources are available to meet necessary obligations and address outstanding issues.

1. Initiatives are listed following a chronological order, when appropriate, or according to their specific relevance to the context discussed in the text.

### *Strategic planning*

The strong engagement of governments is key to maintaining the nuclear knowledge base; sustained government support, policies and clear vision being the most effective means to preserve and grow nuclear knowledge. This needs to be in addition to the role of governments in funding high-risk long-term R&D and ensuring an effective regulator to keep high standards of safety, security and safeguards.

Ten years after the publication of NEA, 2000, most governments appear to have only maintained the *status quo*, with little input at the governmental level in regard to planning for nuclear HR needs. A few, however, have favourably addressed education, human resource capacity and related infrastructure, in some instances marking a real paradigm shift. In some cases this has involved strong co-operation with the industry.

### *Manpower assessments*

As a preliminary step to integrated HR planning, some countries have undertaken manpower assessments. Through comprehensive national surveys, countries such as France, Japan, Korea and the United Kingdom have monitored workforce supply and demand. In some cases, as a result, effective government actions have been triggered to address gaps, including strategic infrastructure planning and provision of financial support.

Over the last decade, the **United Kingdom** government has commissioned various important assessments on the manpower status of the nuclear industry, including, amongst others, the *Study on Nuclear and Radiological Skills*[2] conducted in 2002. One of the principal outcomes of such study was the establishment, around 2003, of Cogent Sector Skills Council to facilitate a demand-led link between government, industry and E&T providers, with the direct involvement of regulators. The key role of Cogent has been to undertake in-depth analyses on the needs of the new build labour market, which have culminated in four "Renaissance" reports[3] assessing the shape of the workforce in the nuclear industry, identifying growth scenarios, the likely demand for skills, potential emerging gaps, and the need for training and qualifications.

Another interesting example is that of **Korea**, where, prompted by a decline of student enrolment and the number of nuclear experts, the government sponsored a specific study on the domestic nuclear manpower status in 2002. Korea is, however, one of the rare examples where commitments for HRD monitoring and planning have been deeply ingrained in government policies and practices for a long time. Since the early years of development of nuclear industry, when the intensive and sustained international co-operation and exchange proved vital for the development of indigenous technology, the Korean government (through the Ministry of Education, Science and Technology) has adopted a very systematic approach in addressing HRD, through the Comprehensive Nuclear Energy Promotion Plan (CNEPP). The CNEPP is developed on a quinquennial basis to define high-level directions and objectives as well as more detailed planning for budget and investment, covering infrastructure and manpower. Other studies are summarised below.

| Country | Assessment and follow-up actions | Year |
|---|---|---|
| United Kingdom | The UK government commissioned various assessments on the manpower status of the nuclear industry, including, amongst others, the "Study on Nuclear and Radiological Skills"[4] in 2002. One of the principal outcomes of such study was the establishment, around 2003, of Cogent Sector Skills Council to facilitate a demand-led link between government, industry and E&T providers, with the direct involvement of regulators. In 2004, Cogent Sector Skills Council set up a Nuclear Employers Steering Group covering all aspects of workforce planning of the nuclear UK sector. | Study released in 2002, 2003, 2004 and subsequent information in 2010 |

2. www.berr.gov.uk/files/file23311.pdf.
3. www.cogent-ssc.com/research/nuclearresearch.php.
4. www.berr.gov.uk/files/file23311.pdf.

| Country | Assessment and follow-up actions | Year |
|---|---|---|
| Japan | Several investigations, including quantitative analyses, roadmaps and HR international evaluations have been conducted by the Nuclear Human Resources Development Council, voluntarily established in 2007 through the co-operation of the Japanese government, industrial and academic entities, and R&D organisations to address mid- and long-term nuclear HRD requirements. | Final report issued in 2010<br>(Council on Nuclear Human Resources Development, 2010) |
| France | A study was commissioned by the government to assess the needs of the specific skills required in higher education *vis-à-vis* the available offer from the existing system and potential deficits.<br>In 2008, following the report and its recommendations, a council was set up, the *Conseil des formations pour l'énergie nucléaire* (CFEN, as the Council was renamed in 2010), to serve as interface between government, industrial actors, academic and research institutions.<br>CFEN conducts systematic examinations of education and training needs, the population of students, the education offer and its adequacy, and on the basis of the assessments it gives recommendations to the Office of Higher Education on the need to open new academic curricula.<br>Recently the *Comité stratégique pour la filière nucléaire* (CSFN) has set up various working groups, dealing also with manpower and a detailed analysis of skills and needs in the nuclear sector at various levels, including for trainers.<br>New programmes have stemmed from this close co-operation, leading to a threefold increase in nuclear graduates at the master level. | Study released in early 2008<br>CFEN established in 2008 |
| Finland | The Finnish Ministry of Trade and Industry published a study on nuclear knowledge management (NEA, 2004). The study, developed with the contribution of all the relevant organisations (the regulator, research centres, universities and power utilities) assessed demand and supply of qualified personnel and identified actions to help maintaining high-level nuclear competence. When, in 2002, the decision to construct a new NPP was taken, power companies and the regulator re-evaluated the situation, initiating together new short-term actions. Thanks to this close collaboration of stakeholders, E&T achieved sufficient capacities to address retirement attrition, which projections of the report had predicted to be very severe (with numbers of retirees expected to double or even triple in the following 5-10 years). | 2000 |

*Recommendation* 2.C (NEA, 2000): Governments should support, on a competitive basis, young students. They should also provide adequate resources for vibrant nuclear research and development programmes including modernisation of facilities.

### *Funding for research and educational resources*

Sustained government efforts to support young students and to fund research, have been reported in a few countries and have proved pivotal in certain cases, as demonstrated in the **United States**. Here, the continuous and stable involvement of federal government and legislators with regulators and universities by means of funding and strong relation based interactions in a non-crisis situation has been fundamental in revitalising educational programmes. The federal government has been very active in providing stewardship support to nuclear education programmes at various levels: graduate, undergraduate, community college, trade schools, etc. Figure 2.1 shows trends in federal (Department of Energy/Nuclear Energy – DOE/NE) investment in universities and student enrolment over the last two decades in the United States. Funding and enrolments are closely linked. Public funding was withdrawn in the 1980s causing a severe decline in nuclear engineering programmes (which halved, going down from 50 to 25), as well as a drastic reduction of university reactors (which dropped to just 25 from the initial 66). Following this critical period, and the issue of the report *Cause for Concern*, federal grants in the nuclear sector were re-established. This proved to be crucially important in attracting growing numbers of students into nuclear engineering. Congress shifted support for student, curriculum development, and new faculty to the US NRC in 2007 and a restructured research funding support from DOE was instituted two years later.[5] In the last three fiscal years (2009-2012) DOE/NE has allocated over USD 170 million for university programmes. The NRC support has remained constant at about USD 25 per year.

5. http://energy.gov/articles/department-energy-issues-funding-opportunity-announcements-enhance-nuclear-energy-education.

**Figure 2.1: Trends in federal investment and in university student enrolment**

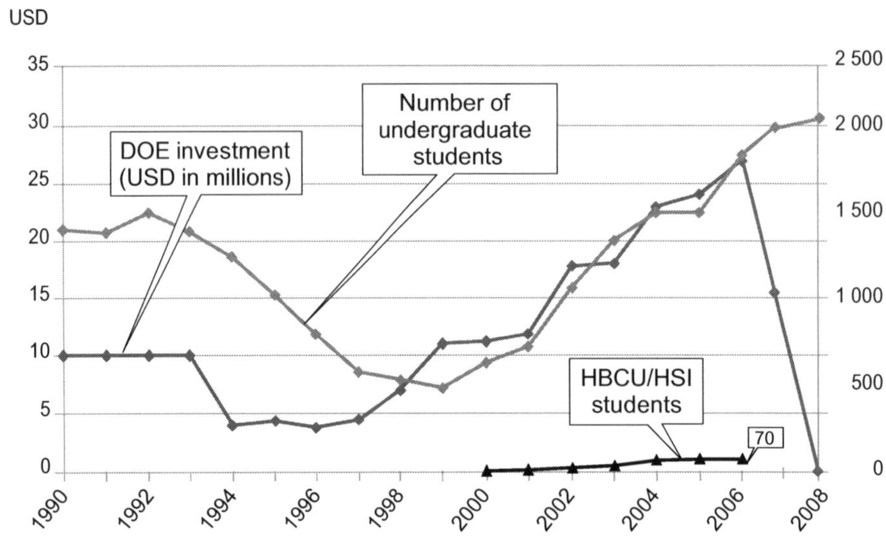


Note: Historically black colleges and universities (HBCUs) are institutions of higher education in the United States that were established before 1964 with the intention of serving the black community. Similarly, HIS are Hispanic-serving institution.

Source: John Gutteridge, Manager, NRC University Programs, presentation to the Nuclear Engineering Department Heads Organisation, American Nuclear Society Annual Meeting, San Diego, CA, 13 June 2010.

Examples of initiatives are given below.

| Country | Funding for research and educational resources | Research/ education |
|---|---|---|
| United States | Government funding of nuclear education can be tied directly to graduation of students focused on nuclear majors. Student interest declined precipitously during the years when government funding for scholarships, fellowships, university research and trade schools was cut. | |
| France | EUR 1 billion have recently been allocated by the government to nuclear research. | Research |
| | In the frame of a 2006 law which sets objectives related to waste management and Generation IV systems, funds were allocated by the government through the national loan *(grand emprunt)*. The ANCRE initiative *(Agence nationale pour la coordination de la recherche sur l'énergie)* coordinates efforts of most French organisations. | |
| | CSFN has also selected R&D strategic targets. Funds for nuclear research have also been raised through different initiatives. | |
| | For education, the government has also allocated grants for students to foster their enrolment (including foreign students, especially in master courses taught in English). | Education |
| Belgium | 45% of the turnover of the Belgian nuclear research centre (SCK•CEN) comes directly from a government grant.<br>Government support to the MYRRHA project with the allocation of EUR 60 million funds over 5 years. | Research |
| Finland | EUR 47 M were allocated in 2007 to fund nuclear research primarily in waste management and reactor safety (on the Finnish Public Research Programme on Nuclear Power Plant Safety – SAFIR). | Research |
| Japan | A programme to sustain universities and colleges in their education plans on nuclear engineering and science was sponsored by the Ministry of Economy, Trading and Industry and the Ministry of Education, Culture, Sports, Science and Technology, in 2007. More than 30 institutions are involved every year (35 universities and 8 colleges in 2010). | Education |

| Country | Funding for research and educational resources | Research/ education |
|---|---|---|
| Korea | Government educational support greatly increased in the last 10 years.<br>Beside the Brain Korea 21st century (BK21) programme started in 1999 by the Ministry of Education, Science and Technology (MEST), the Ministry of Knowledge and Economy (MKE) also established manpower development programmes for industries and universities related to electric industries, with support extended from basic and applied science and engineering research to broader university programmes allowing diversified research, also suited for educational purposes.<br>MEST has provided grants to support research of undergraduate students. Under the programme, started in 2003, ~ 70 to 80 selected students are awarded annually individual research grants of about USD 7 000. The MEST has also provided nuclear E&T grants of USD 0.1 million to each of the eight nuclear engineering departments in Korea.<br>The Nuclear Technology Undergraduate Student Society (NtUss), sponsored by MEST too, has provided its members with a research camp, has organised visits to research institutes and nuclear facilities, lectures and conferences. | Research and education |
| Canada | Government funding for nuclear education and research in universities is partly through the federal Natural Sciences and Engineering Research Council (NSERC). NSERC supports research projects and therefore the development of qualified graduate students. In the nuclear energy field, NSERC generally matches investments made by the nuclear industry.<br>In addition the provincial governments give a per-student grant to their universities in all faculties, including nuclear engineering.<br>Most of the current nuclear R&D in Canada is done by Chalk River Laboratories (CRL), which obtains its funding from both the federal government (for more fundamental research) and nuclear utilities (for R&D relevant to station operating and safety needs). CRL has been a major source of highly qualified personnel (HQP) over the decades. | Research and education |

### *Actions by regulatory authorities*

The nuclear safety authorities have also taken actions, assuming responsibility for issues on national competence in the nuclear sector (NEA, 2004), especially but not exclusively in those cases where direct government initiatives on E&T have been deficient. Such was the case of **Sweden** during the difficult years which followed the phase-out decision, when, in co-operation with the industry (the three nuclear power plants and Westinghouse), the Swedish Nuclear Power Inspectorate set up the Swedish Centre for Nuclear Technology (SKC).[6] SKC's aim was to ensure that nuclear engineering programmes were not completely abandoned at universities and to provide base funding for attractive education and research programmes and their national co-ordination. Initiatives by regulators have also been reported in some other countries:

| Country | Funding for research and educational resources |
|---|---|
| United States | The US NRC has allocated funds for university scholarships and fellowships and faculty development. In 2010, NRC has awarded a total of USD 20 M for its "Education Grant Program", encompassing funds for scholarships and fellowships, faculty development, curriculum development, trade and community college scholarships. NRC has also allocated USD 5 M for the Nuclear Uniform Curriculum Project (see Section 2.2.2). |
| Spain | The Spanish Nuclear Regulatory Body (CSN) has dedicated funds to foster and enhance R&D activities in nuclear safety and radiation protection and to support master courses in nuclear science and technology. CSN has also created and sponsored three chairs in two universities. |
| United Kingdom | At one university, a partnership with the regulatory body and a number of companies has preserved a long-standing nuclear course that would otherwise have closed due to withdrawal of government funding. |

### *Educational networks*

*Recommendation 2.D* (NEA, 2000): Governments should provide support by developing "educational networks or bridges" between universities, industry and research institutes.

6. www.kth.se/sci/centra/skc/aboutus/about-us-1.36901?l=en_UK.

As regards this recommendation, while only feeble indications of progress were reported up to 2004 (NEA, 2004), in recent years an upsurge of educational networks has been registered, at the national and international level. The establishment of such networks and bridges has generally been the result of concerted efforts of different stakeholders: governments, through their support and even, in some instances, their leadership; academic and research institutes, through the joint promotion and co-ordination of nuclear education and R&D programmes; and, not least, the industry. Industry involvement has occurred through financial aid, granting of access to its research facilities for exercises and training and the participation of professionals in the development and delivery of courses, which also facilitates transfer of tacit knowledge (IAEA, 2011).

Noteworthy is also the recent establishment at a European level of the European Nuclear Education Network (ENEN) and the European Nuclear Energy Leadership Academy (ENELA), discussed in later sections.

The development of networks and consortia has been very much in line with the other recommendation raised in the 2000 OECD/NEA report that:

*Recommendation* 4.C (NEA, 2000): Industry, research institutes and universities need to work together to co-ordinate efforts better to encourage the younger generation.

As actions related to Recommendations 2.D and 4.C are closely linked, they are discussed jointly herewith.

In **Canada**, although human resource planning is, to a large extent, the responsibility of the individual organisations (utility, design, research), a significant role in the development and supply of highly qualified personnel has been played since 2002 by the University Network of Excellence in Nuclear Engineering (UNENE).[7] This notable example of cross-collaboration was founded as a non-profit organisation with the support of the government and the nuclear industry (utilities and design organisations) and embraces 12 universities, nuclear federal agencies and nuclear industrial organisations including operators, designers and the regulator. UNENE currently supports seven industrial research chairs in various universities in areas related to nuclear power, as well as several collaborative R&D projects. It also sponsors and co-ordinates a Master of Engineering degree jointly offered by member universities. To help achieving UNENE's goals, the industry is investing significant funds in selected universities and is contributing in-kind to enable universities to acquire and retain the highest quality of teaching and research professoriate. The universities secure additional funds from NSERC and elsewhere, to match investments made by the nuclear industry. All the major organisations, which run training programmes for in-house staff, have also donated much of their material to UNENE as a supplemental resource for the UNENE, its professors and students. In 2007-2009, the UNENE investment in nuclear research was instrumental in the successful award of research grants. Other networks established in the last decade are outlined below.

| Country | Network | Year of creation |
|---|---|---|
| Belgium | BNEN: Belgian Nuclear Higher Education Network<br>*Objectives:* to maintain and further develop a high quality programme in nuclear engineering, to remodel nuclear education in Belgium, catalysing networks between academia, research centres and public utilities<br>*Membership:* founded by SCK•CEN and five Belgian universities with the sponsorship of the Belgian nuclear industries – a sixth university joined the programme in the academic year 2006-2007.<br>*Achievements:* "Master after Master" instituted from the amalgamation of different programmes into a single nuclear programme for holders of a master degree in engineering. Highly modular and taught in English. | 2001 |

7. www.unene.ca/.

| Country | Network | Year of creation |
|---|---|---|
| Japan | JN-HRD Net: Japan Nuclear Human Resource Development Network<br>*Objectives:* to co-ordinate effort in inter-sector activities for education and training of students, young researchers and engineers, in line with the proposals of the Nuclear HRD Council.<br>*Membership:* initiated by the government involving academic institutions, industries, public bodies and R&D organisations – 62 participating organisations as of summer 2011.<br>*Initiatives:* establishment of the University Union, a university network including the Tokyo Institute of Technology and 14 universities and co-ordinating new education programmes for their students and internationally. | |
| | JNEN: Japan Nuclear Education Network<br>Established by the Japan Atomic Energy Agency (JAEA) and three universities and now extended to six participating universities. | 2007 |
| | *Other educational networks:*<br>Regional activities supported by local governments e.g. the joint project promoted by the Prefecture of Fukui (counting 13 NPPs and the fast breeder reactor Monju). Supported by local governments, it benefits from the co-operation utility companies, universities, manufacturers and JAEA, capitalising on the experience of nuclear organisations to provide E&T nationally and for the Asian region. | |
| Finland | FINNEN: Finnish Nuclear Education Network<br>Driven by the government. FINNEN offers several courses at Lappeenranta University and Helsinki University of Technology (EC, 2009). | |
| United Kingdom | NTEC: Nuclear Technology Education Consortium<br>Created between universities and other institutions to provide postgraduate nuclear education.<br>Many other industry-university consortia have also been created, such as the Nuclear Academic Industry Liaison Sub Committee of the Nuclear Institute (NAILs). | |
| Germany | Alliance for Competence in Nuclear Technology (in German: *Kompetenzverbund Kerntechnik*)<br>Involving the combined effort of research centres, the nuclear industry, universities and the government.<br>Other associations oriented either towards regional needs or related to specific technical areas were formed in the following years and include:<br>– the South-western Nuclear Research and Education Alliance;<br>– the Western Nuclear Forum; the Competence Alliance of Radiation Research; and<br>– the Repository Research Group.<br>Objectives: the identification of future needs on nuclear HR and capacity for E&T, the enhanced collaboration between universities and international networks, the co-ordination of projects for nuclear safety and waste management R&D, the promotion of young nuclear scientists and engineers, the participation in further developments of international nuclear standards. | 2000 |
| Italy | CIRTEN: *Consorzio Interuniversitario per la Ricerca Tecnologica Nucleare*<br>Founded by the seven Italian "nuclear universities" with the aim of promoting nuclear scientific and technological research and co-ordinating the development of nuclear knowledge and collaboration with national and international research institutions and industries.<br>ANIMP: *Associazione Nazionale Impiantistica Industriale*<br>Plays a role of co-ordination of industries and utilities. It has recently launched the Executive Master in Nuclear Plant Construction Management, in collaboration with universities (and in particular the *Politectico di Milano*). | 1994 |

Sometimes supported by the government, partnerships between academic and research institutions with the industry have helped establishing new courses, as exemplified below and in Section 2.2.2. Raising the profile of research in the nuclear area through the formation of industry-university research alliances sometimes has enhanced the interest in nuclear subjects among undergraduates, as in the United Kingdom, where students are also attracted by the prospect of new build. The result has been a net increase in the number of students attending existing nuclear options and the introduction of new ones.

| Country | New courses and educational schemes established through the collaborative effort of different stakeholders |
|---|---|
| Switzerland | Swiss NE Master: Swiss Master of Science in Nuclear Engineering established in 2008<br>Essentially due to self-generated motivation at the academic level, involving the Swiss Federal Institutes of Technology (EPFL at Lausanne and ETHZ at Zurich) and the Paul Scherrer Institute (PSI) at Villigen, as national research centre, and Swissnuclear, the association of Swiss nuclear utilities. Contributions from the nuclear industry to the Swiss NE Master include the provision of lecturers in several courses and the offer of industrial internships to the students. The industry has also been financing nearly 50% of the R&D activities of PSI's Nuclear Energy and Safety (NES) department. A part of the financial support is separately earmarked for PhD students and young scientists. |
| Japan | Collaboration between different academic institutions and the industry is well established in Japan: lectures and practical exercises are conducted with the participation of utilities, manufacturers and JAEA at universities willing to run nuclear related courses but lacking professional staff.<br>The Professional School of Nuclear Engineering of the University of Tokyo is operated in co-operation with JAEA, which provides more than 70 experts (researchers and engineers) as visiting professors or lecturers every year, with more than 90% of experimental exercises conducted at JAEA research facilities (including accelerators, neutron irradiation facilities, etc., and various reactors). |
| United Kingdom | The "Nuclear Graduates Scheme" was set up with the support of the government and 20 leading companies and organisations operating in the United Kingdom nuclear industry. Hosted by the Nuclear Decommissioning Authority (NDA), this highly selective nuclear graduate programme offers a breadth of technical experience from across government sites, supply chain and regulators, providing also subsequent placement opportunities in the industry. |

### 2.2.2 University initiatives

*Recommendation* 3.A (NEA, 2000): Universities should provide basic and attractive educational programmes.

While some countries have experienced challenges in maintaining national education and training infrastructure (in particular those with declining nuclear programmes or where smaller numbers of specialists are required) the general outlook of nuclear academic programmes seems to have improved over the last ten years. Some new and advanced nuclear courses are being launched in an increasingly global context. And these have sometimes succeeded attracting healthier numbers of students, whose interest may be stimulated by the prospect of new build, or high profile research topics and international projects.

In **Sweden**, nuclear education has now reached a very good state, with the numbers of students and professors markedly on the increase. Different education programmes are active in universities at various levels. Numerous new academic activities have also recently started, including the first dedicated programme in nuclear engineering at bachelor level, just launched in the autumn of 2010 at Uppsala University; the new nuclear engineering MSc started in the autumn 2009 by the Chalmers Institute of Technology, in Gothenburg, to train specialists for the nearby nuclear power plants.

Other examples of emerging programmes are shown below.

| Country | Examples of emerging university programmes |
|---|---|
| France | Comprehensive, diversified and more specialised nuclear-related engineering programmes are provided in more than 30 engineering schools and universities through a well established and robust nuclear education system. Some longstanding and other recently launched courses, covering core and nuclear engineering disciplines as well as more specific subjects (e.g. chemistry/cycle or materials for nuclear/fuel, or safety/security, or cleaning and dismantling) offer a growing supply capacity. In the last four years enrolment of students at master level or equivalent has increased from less than 300 to approximately 900 students for the year 2009-2010, and to 1 000 for the year 2010-2011. Recruitment of teachers has also expanded.<br>Most of the nuclear specialised curricula last 1 or 2 years. |
| Japan | Introduction of new nuclear education programmes for graduate students, including those under the University Union and some more unconventional courses, e.g. on "nuclear energy sociology" taught at the University of Tokyo and covering three major "social-related" subjects: nuclear law and regulation, nuclear non-proliferation and the harmonisation of society and nuclear technology. |

| Country | Examples of emerging university programmes |
|---|---|
| Canada | Specialised programmes provided by the University of Ontario Institute of Technology (UOIT) and McMaster University for students who want to improve their knowledge in specific areas and in a shorter period of time. Good rate of undergraduate enrolment of 250 and 35 students respectively in Nuclear Engineering and in Health Physics and Radiation Science at UOIT. |
| Spain | New advanced courses have been set up in some universities over and above basic, more traditional nuclear subjects, and include: transmutation, material science, advanced computer codes, nuclear fusion technology, etc. These topics sought by the sector are appealing to students.<br>In 2011, the Polytechnical University of Catalonia launched a new Master in Nuclear Technology,[8] taught in English, in collaboration with one of the Spanish utilities (ENDESA). |
| Belgium | Four-year master courses in nuclear technology, medical nuclear techniques and radiochemistry organised by three Belgian institutes.<br>Radiation Protection Expert course granting the qualification of "radiation expert" started by SCK•CEN, two Belgian technical universities together with IRE *(Institut National des Radio-Éléments)*. |
| Italy | Two new master courses have started in the Universities of Bologna (2008) and Genoa (2010), the latter partially founded by the European Union (EU). The master degree in nuclear safety and security delivered at the University of Pisa with the collaborative effort of industry, research centres and institutions (e.g. CIRTEN, Ansaldo Nucleare, ITER Consult, etc.) provides a curriculum in nuclear safety and security compatible with other nuclear engineering programmes in Europe. This is preceded by a preparatory course for students with MSc in industrial and civil engineering, but also physics and chemistry, to have a basic formation in nuclear science and technology. |
| United Kingdom | At the master level, British universities have preserved existing courses, and introduced new ones, as a result of discussions with the industry and in response to identified needs (see also Section 2.2.1). |

Some other countries have experienced an upturn in student enrolment, such as in the **United States**, where, as already mentioned above, the declining trend seen in nuclear education during the 1980s and 1990s has decidedly reversed since the year 2000. A positive trend that can be ascribed to new important university programmes and courses as well the establishment of inter-university consortia and college partnerships; advancements which have largely been possible thanks to the very sizeable allocation of federal funds.

In **Germany,** education, especially at postgraduate levels, has been enhanced by coupling with attractive research topics and international collaboration projects. Interestingly, the number of professors at universities has seen a considerable rise in recent years up to 2010, in contrast to the previous forecast made in 2004.[9]

*Recommendation* 3.B (NEA, 2000): Universities should interact early and often with potential students, both male and female, and provide adequate information.

It is important that universities inform and encourage prospective students to choose nuclear related courses. As a recent survey conducted in **Switzerland** by Nuklearforum Schweiz[10] has shown, pre-university students are much more open to the notion of nuclear energy as part of a sustainable energy mix than are their school teachers.

In some countries universities are engaging with technical colleges, sometimes franchising courses and establishing partnerships to address the increasing demand of craft and technical levels in the sector (as discussed in Section 2.2.6).

Initiatives are taken in this respect by various universities, for instance through the organisation of summer schools or "mentor projects" to give secondary school students an insight into nuclear courses (NEA, 2004).

8. http://formaciocontinua.upc.edu/nuclearengineering.

9. Statistics indicated that there were 20 professors in nuclear education in 2010, a much healthier figure than what trends derived from the survey in 2000 and 2002/2004 had predicted, according to which, in 2010, respectively 10 and 5 nuclear professorships were expected to remain active.

10. www.nuklearforum.ch.

In **Japan**, some universities foster nuclear subjects in their neighbouring schools; others open up lectures to the public (NEA, 2004).

### *2.2.3 Industry initiatives*

*Recommendation* 4.A (NEA, 2000): Industry should continue to provide rigorous training programmes to meet its specific needs.

*Recommendation* 4.C (NEA, 2000): Industry, research institutes and universities need to work together to co-ordinate efforts better to encourage the younger generation (discussed above).

The industry has generally kept playing a key role in actively monitoring HRD demand and supply and in providing high-quality, in-house training (of course not for academic credit) of their nuclear power plant staff.

In many companies, HRD is still done in house, with a big part performed through "on-the-job training" within individual facilities, trying to ensure the transfer of technical knowledge from the more experienced to younger personnel. Most utility companies conduct personnel's training through systematic programmes and dedicated equipment, such as large scale nuclear power plant operation simulators. This is the case of utilities in the **United States**, where all power reactors have large full scale reactor simulators, but some utilities are exploring the possibilities of utilising research reactors to enhance training of reactor fundamentals for engineers and other plant workers who need to understand such basic nuclear phenomena as reactivity feedback and control. Equally, in **Japan**, collaboration is often sought with universities and R&D organisations, such as JAEA.

| Country | Industry initiatives |
|---|---|
| France | AREVA[11] has recently taken very decisive actions with its training programmes to satisfy its high and diverse recruitment needs and also to provide solutions for nuclear training and the enhancement of all nuclear related skills to its partners, customers and suppliers. Both *Électricité de France* (EDF)[12] and GDF SUEZ[13] run their own established training programmes, combining courses with job training and covering topics which range from nuclear fundamentals to safety and focus not only on scientific and technical subjects, but also on project management. For their newly engaged engineers GDF SUEZ organises a one-year training in **Belgium**, with courses provided also by SCK•CEN. |
| Korea | Korea Hydro & Nuclear Power (KHNP) expanded its own manpower development process to include a mid- and long-term training and education programmes for its employees. The courses (about 150) consist of internal and external training programmes and include also management and leadership courses. |
| United Kingdom | In 2005, Atkins founded the Nuclear Academy, a training institution for its employees, and in 2008, with the same intention, British Energy created the Nuclear Power Academy. Nuclear industry supports the Cogent National Occupational Standards, National Vocational Qualifications and Foundation Degrees.<br>As discussed earlier, 20 leading companies and organisations operating in the United Kingdom nuclear industry has contributed in setting up the "Nuclear Graduates Scheme". |
| Spain | HR needs for the domestic industry have been satisfied so far and new training programmes are being set up, notably by the engineering companies Tecnatom, and *Empresarios Agrupados* (EA), and by *Centro de Investigaciones Energéticas, Medioambientales y Tecnológicas* (CIEMAT). The nuclear industry is enhancing activities of R&D through the CEYDEN Platform. |

A serious challenge faced by the nuclear industry, and, in particular, some of its specific sectors, is (non-retirement) attrition: external attrition with other industries such as oil and gas, as well as internal attrition. This issue is quite critical in the United Kingdom, where the decommissioning supply chain competes for talent with a build-out programme, but it could become important also in other countries.

A noteworthy example of industrial co-operation is the Center for Energy Workforce Development (CEWD) established in 2006 in the **United States** as a non-profit consortium of indus-

11. www.areva.com.
12. www.edf.fr.
13. www.gdfsuez.com.

tries: electric, natural gas and nuclear energy utilities and their associations, in collaboration with Nuclear Energy Institute (NEI). Through this concerted effort of different sectors CEWD aims at helping energy utilities work together to develop solutions to an expected workforce shortage during the coming decades.

As well as training, sometimes industry has been highly engaged with education programmes by funding chairs, sponsoring educational programmes, developing and delivering courses, offering internships and, in some cases, opening infrastructure to students (e.g. for the preparation of theses). This has already been discussed in Section 2.2.1 and is further exemplified below.

| Country | Initiative |
|---|---|
| France | Chairs in schools and universities are funded by the industry.<br>In 2008, EDF allocated EUR 4 million to set up the *"Fondation européenne pour les énergies de demain"* in collaboration with the *Institut de France* to fund higher education projects and research in clean energies and subsidise student grants. |
| Sweden | The industry is involved both as sponsors and as contributors with teachers in the delivery of education programmes. Together with the regulatory body, industry contributes to the funding of the already mentioned Swedish Nuclear Technology Centre in order to ensure that there is adequate financial provision to replace retiring professors (NEA, 2004).<br>The industrial full-scale reactor simulators are also made available for student training. All Swedish universities have bilateral collaborations with industries and, typically, the nuclear power plants support the geographically closest university. |
| Switzerland | The industry has been supporting the Chair in Nuclear Energy Systems at the Swiss Federal Institute of Technology in Zurich, after the university decided in 2004 to suppress its Chair in Nuclear Engineering. |
| Germany | Co-operation between the industry and educational institutions, in particular at PhD level, has been strengthened. In collaboration with research institutions and universities, some German nuclear industries finance young scientists' research work on their PhD theses. Nuclear industries such as EnBW and AREVA, have also sponsored professorships at German universities, a significant contribution to enhance nuclear education in Germany. |
| Finland | Summer training periods in industries are compulsory and students have been able to work with the industry, research institutes and nuclear authorities to prepare their theses. |

Aspects such as **career development and continuous professional training, retention and development of competencies and skills** are also central aspects of HRD for those in employment in the nuclear sector. Succession planning is of prime importance in the nuclear industry. Many companies invest in knowledge management systems, usually as a way of retaining information as experienced staff leave (NEA, 2004). In addition, the participation of industry professionals in the development and delivery of courses at educational programmes is certainly beneficial in this respect, as it allows the transfer of implicit or tacit knowledge as well as explicit knowledge (IAEA, 2011).

Smaller companies and subcontractors often have a difficult time structuring training programmes and the **use of outside companies to help deliver training** has become a practice adopted quite commonly (see also Chapter 3). In **Finland,** FinNuclear[14] was established in 2009 to provide training for potential subcontractors organising and co-ordinating all-around training, education and networking for the Finnish Suppliers Group members. **In Sweden** (KSU, 2009), the nuclear training and safety centre KSU, part of the Vattenfall Group and owned by the industry, provides training and measures to develop staff skills for the Swedish nuclear power industry, according to their short- and long-term needs. The company also produces and manages educational material needed for its training activities. Also, in **Spain,** training is outsourced to specialised organisations and engineering firms; here TECNATOM, *Empresarios Agrupados* and CIEMAT are setting up new training programmes.

14. www.prizz.fi/sivu.aspx?taso=1&id=392.

### *Role of nuclear societies*

Active scientific and learned societies play a positive role in E&T in several countries. Such is the case of **Spain**, where the Foro of the Nuclear Industry and the Spanish Nuclear Society have co-ordinated efforts towards the dissemination of information on nuclear energy and its advantages in intermediate and high schools to professors and students. The Foro has organised E&T programmes, such as the Basic Course on Nuclear Energy, and seminars in the whole national territory; it has promoted summer schools for young university students in collaboration with *Universidad Politécnica de Madrid* (UPM) and granted scholarships and prizes to young students.

More examples are provided below.

| Country | Initiatives by nuclear societies |
|---|---|
| Japan | In 2005 a senior network activity in the Atomic Energy Society of Japan was started by some retired experts. The experts are voluntarily creating opportunities to talk directly to the young generation, mostly university students in fields not related to nuclear. More than 30 meetings have been organised between 2005 and 2009. |
| Korea | In Korea, the NtUss sponsored by MEST has provided its members with a research camp, organised visits to research institutes and nuclear facilities as well as lectures and conferences, designed to give the next generations an overall picture and experiences of the nuclear society and to promote networking (NEA, 2004). |
| United Kingdom | In 2009, the British Nuclear Energy Society[15] and the Institution of Nuclear Engineers merged together in the Nuclear Institute (NI) that represents nuclear professionals in the United Kingdom. NI fosters activities for the advancement of nuclear science, engineering and technology, and more specifically for maintaining high standards of education and professional performance amongst engineers, scientists and others working within the nuclear industry. It also promotes public understanding of nuclear sciences. |
| United States | The American Nuclear Society has 10 000 members. They co-ordinate dozens of conferences and topical meeting annually to help further nuclear science and technology research. Every year they host a student based conference for the nuclear engineering programmes. This conference provides a venue for nuclear engineering students to present their research. The 2011 conference had over 670 attendees including 505 students and 165 student presentations. In 1999, North American Young Generation in Nuclear and a US chapter of Women in Nuclear were established. These organisations now represent nearly 13 000 professionals working in all segments of nuclear science and technology. They organise annual workshops aimed at helping members in their professional development. |

### *2.2.4 Research institute initiatives*

*Recommendation* 4.B (NEA, 2000): Research institutes need to develop exciting research projects to meet industry's needs and attract quality students and employees.

In most countries research institutes have made efforts to promote high profile research projects and co-ordinate with universities and other stakeholders, e.g. through the promotion and delivery of courses and seminars to a varied audience, the offer of internships, the provision of well-equipped laboratories and guidance to domestic and foreign students for their research, the award of prizes, grants and fellowships, the organisation of visits, etc. These activities bring undergraduate and graduate students into contact with the research institutes in a manner that can only encourage employment in the industry if not the research institute itself (NEA, 2004). Opening the facilities to visits is an effective way of prompting the dissemination of factual information on nuclear technology, which helps developing a better understanding and, triggering interest amongst the public and students.

Some prominent examples of different initiatives by research institutes are briefly discussed below. An appraisal of the use of research facilities for education and training purposes is provided in Section 2.3.

15. www.nuclearinst.com/ibis/Nuclear%20Institute/Home.


NUCLEAR EDUCATION AND TRAINING: FROM CONCERN TO CAPABILITY, ISBN 978-92-64-17637-9, © OECD 2012

| Country | Examples of research institutions initiatives and their support to educational programmes |
|---|---|
| France | Scientific co-operation is being enhanced, especially within the French Alternative Energies and Atomic Energy Commission (*Commission à l'énergie atomique et aux énergies alternatives* – CEA), the Institute for Radiation Protection and Nuclear Safety (*Institut de radioprotection et de sûreté nucléaire* – IRSN) and the National Center for Scientific Research (*Centre national de la recherché scientifique* – CNRS) as well as amongst university laboratories. Opportunities are offered to students for the preparation of theses: the CEA welcomes PhD students and trainees in its research and development laboratories where they can develop their research on numerous R&D topics and often in tight co-operation with industry. This has led to the doubling of the number of PhD students during the last five years. The IRSN[16] is in charge of the training of medical personnel and other workers exposed to radiation in the workplace and provides a wide range of advanced training sessions in nuclear safety and regulation, as well as initial training in radiation protection. Together with other European Technical Safety Organisation (TSOs), IRSN has created a professional training institute in the field of nuclear safety, the European Nuclear Safety Training and Tutoring Institute (ENSTTI),[17] to design new training programmes aiming, in the first instance, to establish a common culture in nuclear risk assessment amongst regulators and TSOs within Europe.<br>Experts from R&D organisations contribute to various academic curricula throughout France in the frame of strategic partnerships. Through the National Institute for Nuclear Science and Technology (INSTN), CEA provides technicians, engineers and researchers with highly specialised courses in nuclear science and technology, including graduate-level curricula. Today the INSTN offers a selection of nearly 210 continuing education sessions from its catalogue or on demand, some of which in English. INSTN also participates in the "train the teachers and instructors" programme created in 2009. |
| Japan | JAEA, the largest organisation for R&D on nuclear technology conducts a wide variety of training courses for engineers and scientists, seminars for government and local government officers, and educational activities for the public. This is carried out through its Nuclear Human Resource Development Centre.<br>JAEA has also strong collaboration with universities and professional schools, holding co-operative agreements with 20 academic institutions.<br>As mentioned, JAEA collaborates with the University of Tokyo in operation of the Professional School of Nuclear Engineering founded in 2005 and JAEA has also helped connecting several universities through JNEN and its Internet-based platform. |
| Korea | The Korea Atomic Energy Research Institute (KAERI) provides an extensive in-house E&T programme, including fundamental and advanced courses for its own members, as industry personnel and university students. Practical and managerial courses, including research reactor training for undergraduate students in nuclear engineering and web-based E&T programmes are delivered.<br>University research grants are on the increase and graduate students participate in R&D projects run by KAERI and the Korea Institute for Nuclear Safety (KINS), fostering the development of the next generation of researchers and enhancing the co-ordination of research projects between research institutes and universities.<br>The Korea Nuclear Foundation (KNEF) holds a nuclear facility visit programme for undergraduate students which count as part of the course about 100 students participate every year.<br>Longstanding internship programmes in research institutes and industrial organisations often lead to employment. Due to the limited resources, joint research initiatives among industries, universities and research organisations have been particularly beneficial in Korea, allowing the development of original and self-reliant technologies. |
| Spain | CIEMAT and the Institute of Nuclear Fusion at UPM, have been very active in high profile research programmes, as well as E&T activities in collaboration with universities and international research centres.<br>The National Technology Platform for Nuclear Fission Energy R&D – *Plataforma Tecnológica de Energía Nuclear de Fisión* (CEIDEN)[18] was created in 2007 to co-ordinate the needs and efforts of the Spanish R&D in the field of fission nuclear technology.<br>Within this framework a one-year Master in Nuclear Technology and Applications (MINA) has been established in 2008 by CIEMAT, with the collaboration of several universities, the support of the nuclear industry and the participation of an increasing number of students from Spain as well as South America. |
| Switzerland | PSI has been instrumental in supporting educational needs. It is here that most of the nuclear fission related PhD research is conducted – largely in the framework of collaborations with the two Swiss Federal Institutes of Technology.<br>Since 2008, with the establishment of the Swiss Master of Science in Nuclear Engineering, PSI has also been hosting the corresponding master thesis projects. |

16. www.irsn.fr.
17. www.enstti.eu.
18. www.ceiden.com.

| Country | Examples of research institutions initiatives and their support to educational programmes |
|---|---|
| United Kingdom | After years with no national nuclear research institute, the National Nuclear Laboratory[19] was established to provide leading nuclear technology services through technical innovation and intellectual support, including: helping to reduce the cost of clean-up and decommissioning, maintaining critical skills, attracting new people to the industry, and working with cognate organisations around the world. However, its funding remains uncertain.<br>In addition, building on existing partnerships with EDF Energy, Rolls-Royce and AWE, the new Nuclear Research Centre (NRC), a joint venture between the University of Bristol and the University of Oxford, has officially been opened in late 2011 to help developing a skilled workforce for the UK's nuclear industry. The new centre aims at providing leading edge and innovative research to support the design and safe operation of current and future generations of nuclear systems, including both fundamental research and work on emergent topics.<br>Separately, the Nuclear Advanced Manufacturing Research Centre has been created as a joint venture between the universities of Manchester and Sheffield. |
| Belgium | SCK•CEN's Academy for Nuclear Science and Technology co-ordinates and organises training programmes for professionals in various topics covered in its research remit, with the prime objective of gathering and spreading the necessary knowledge in the nuclear field.<br>There are many links between SCK•CEN and academic institutions. SCK•CEN offers internships, hires and provides guidance to PhD candidates and postdoctoral researchers, awarding prizes to the best master theses (NEA, 2004). Some SCK•CEN experts have also professorships at universities where they teach modules in regular academic programmes.<br>Pupils from the last year of high school have the possibility to visit SCK•CEN and talk with its experts monthly. |
| Sweden | Sweden closed its research reactors a few years ago. Transnational training exercises are organised in the TRIGA reactor in Helsinki. Ferries frequently cross the Baltic Sea and part of the courses are taught onboard at the conference facilities of these ships.<br>BR1 at SCK•CEN in Belgium and the training reactor at Budapest University of Technology and Economics have also been used. |

### 2.2.5 International organisation initiatives

A plethora of organisations exist to support the nuclear industry at various levels of educational, professional, trade, governmental organisation, etc. This section reviews those whose origins are intergovernmental or corporate international and whose scope includes internationalisation in education, training or knowledge management. Excluded for these reasons are the initiatives of trade associations and learned societies.

The principal agents in this area are: the IAEA, the OECD/NEA and the pan-European initiatives of the European Commission and Euratom. The following extracts represent a selection from the many initiatives that have emerged over the last decade. Further details on each are best reviewed from the websites of the respective organisation.

#### *The International Atomic Energy Agency*

It is set out in the statute mandates of the IAEA that the Agency foster the exchange of scientific and technical information and encourage exchange in the education and training of scientists and experts in the field of peaceful uses of atomic energy.[20] To this end, very significant resources have been allocated by the Agency for activities supporting nuclear education and training over the last decade. Of particular note in this regard are the Nuclear Knowledge Management unit (NKM)[21] and the Nuclear Power Engineering Section (NPES).[22]

The main objectives of NKM are to assess the status of and trends in nuclear education, including the harmonisation of curricula in nuclear education and the preservation of knowledge. In discharging this responsibility, the NKM initiative faces both the newcomer nation with nuclear energy capacity programmes, as well as the mature with established programmes.

19. www.nnl.co.uk/.
20. www.iaea.org/About/statute_text.html.
21. www.iaea.org/inisnkm/nkm/index.html.
22. www.iaea.org/NuclearPower/Engineering/about.html.

For the newcomer nation, capacity building through training, education and transferring knowledge are key to acquiring the skilled human resources to design, build and operate nuclear installations. For the established programme, securing a skilled supply of human resources is required to sustain the safe operation of existing installations, their decommissioning and related programmes for spent fuel and waste as well as support for new build in those countries willing to pursue it.

NKM is also developing methodologies and guidance for the international community including the evaluation and benchmarking of national nuclear education programmes together with knowledge management.

The NKM organises activities, events, resources and issues publications.

❑ Activities

Methodology and guidance, e.g. the Assist Mission and the Nuclear Energy Handbook.

The former involves disseminating good practice and making recommendations for improvement; the latter is a growing database of annotated weblinks in the fields of nuclear science and technology.

Expert bodies and networks that facilitate sustainable education and training. Of particular note are the:

- World Nuclear University[23] (in partnership with other organisations – as discussed in Section 2.2.6);
- School of Nuclear Energy Management;
- School of Nuclear Knowledge Management;
- Asian Network for Education in Nuclear Training (ANENT);
- African Regional Co-operative Agreement for Research, Development;
- Regional Co-operative Agreement for Research, Development and Training Related to Nuclear Science and Technology for Asia and the Pacific.

Supporting knowledge maintenance, analysis and integration, mainly in fast reactors together with a nuclear archive.

Providing assistance and services to NPPs and other nuclear installations, including workshops on human resource management.

Other activities, such as the global NPP survey: *Investigating the Link between Knowledge Management Practices and Organisational Performance.*[24]

❑ Resources

A gateway to scientific and technical knowledge, as well as guidance to member states, including:

Publications[25] such as, among others:

- *Status and Trends in Nuclear Education* (IAEA, 2011);
- *Workforce Planning for New Nuclear Power Programmes* (IAEA, 2011a);
- *Development of Knowledge Portals for Nuclear Power Plants* (IAEA, 2009);
- *Managing Human Resources in the Field of Nuclear Energy* (IAEA, 2009a);
- *Milestones in the Development of a National Infrastructure for Nuclear Power* (IAEA, 2007);
- *Competency Assessments for Nuclear Industry Personnel* (IAEA, 2006).

23. www.world-nuclear-university.org/.
24. www.iaea.org/inisnkm/nkm/global_NPP_Survey.html.
25. For a comprehensive catalogue of NKM publications, see: http://iaea.org/inisnkm/nkm/nkmPublications.html.

Databases. A resource of more than 20 databases, including International Nuclear Information System (INIS), a world's largest collection of "grey" literature on the peaceful uses of nuclear science and technology.

Directories, such as the aforementioned Nuclear Energy Handbook and worldwide listings.

- ☐ Events

A comprehensive annual programme of events, including provision for the School of Nuclear Energy Management and outputs of regional networks (initiatives already mentioned above), together with the dissemination of good practice and e-learning platforms.[26]

In addition to the activities of the NKM unit, the NPES includes in its remit guidance and proven practices pertaining to:

- attitudes and professionalism of NPP personnel;
- effective methods for NPP personnel training;
- training and performance of NPP contractors;
- training for the commissioning of NPPs;
- knowledge management and quality management of NPP training programmes.

The global Nuclear Power Human Resource Survey[27] has been recently launched under the auspices of NPES.

In addition to its own programme of activities, the NPES is also a portal to activities and publications such as those identified under NKM.

Other IAEA initiatives worthy of note are in the area of nuclear security. The IAEA has taken the lead to develop, together with academics and experts from member states, a technical guidance for a Master of Science programme and a certificate programme (IAEA, 2010a). The International Nuclear Security Education Network (INSEN) was also established as a partnership between the IAEA, educational and research institutions and other stakeholders with the mission of enhancing global nuclear security by developing, sharing and promoting excellence in nuclear security education. At this stage, the INSEN membership (currently comprising 45 members and four observers) is informal and open to any educational and research institution already running or planning nuclear security education programmes.

*The OECD Nuclear Energy Agency*

As a prime international organisation in the field of nuclear energy, the OECD/NEA has a role to focus directly on E&T as part of nuclear development, regulation and operation, being also able to maintain a unique capability in knowledge management. OECD/NEA committees have different emphases and outcomes of their respective work include review reports on the status across NEA member countries, statements (including the 2007 Statement by the OECD/NEA Steering Committee – NEA, 2007), specialist courses (e.g. in nuclear law), specialist reports on specific aspects (e.g. R&D facilities, such as NEA, 2009 and NEA, 2009a), compilation and management of databanks bringing together collective experience from many countries, joint programmes among regulators, waste operators, etc. The flagship publication *Cause for Concern?* (NEA, 2000) issued under the auspices of the OECD/NEA Committee for Technical and Economic Studies on Nuclear Energy Development and the Fuel Cycle has been amply discussed in this report, together with its follow-up study NEA (2004).

26. e.g. www.iaea.org/inisnkm/nkm/e_learning/index.htm.
27. http://iaeaglobalworkforce.org/survey/workforcesurvey.asp.

A synopsis of some of the other specific activities carried out within different OECD/NEA divisions over the last 10 years is provided below.

| Division | Initiative |
|---|---|
| Nuclear Development | *Nuclear Education and Training: Cause for Concern?* (2000) (already discussed)<br>*Nuclear Competence Building* (2004) (already discussed) |
| Legal Affairs | *International School of Nuclear Law*<br>The International School of Nuclear Law (ISNL), established in 2001 by the NEA in co-operation with the University of Montpellier 1, is designed to provide participants with a comprehensive understanding of the various interrelated legal issues governing the safe, efficient and secure use of nuclear energy. The programme has evolved over the last decade to address developments in nuclear law. To date, the ISNL has provided a unique educational opportunity to more than 600 graduate students and young professionals from around the world. Participants have the possibility to apply for a University Diploma in International Nuclear Law from the University of Montpellier, recognised within the ECTS (European Credit Transfer and Accumulation System).<br>*International Nuclear Law Essentials*<br>The five-day International Nuclear Law Essentials (INLE) course, first held in October 2011, provides participants with a comprehensive understanding of the various interrelated legal issues on the safe, efficient and secure use of nuclear energy. This intensive course has been designed to accommodate the needs and interests of mid-career lawyers working in either the public or the private sector, and is also of interest to scientists, policy-makers and managers. A certificate of completion is conferred by the NEA at the end of the course.<br>*Other*<br>NEA Legal Affairs engages in various other activities to provide and promote educational opportunities in the nuclear field:<br>• It maintains information regarding educational opportunities in the nuclear field on its website.[28]<br>• Legal experts from NEA Legal Affairs have lectured at various events, conferences and symposia that draw an international audience (e.g. the WNU, and the International Nuclear Law course sponsored by the International Center of the Lomonosov Moscow State University). |
| Data Bank | The Data Bank has 50 years of experience in generating, gathering, exchanging, distributing and preserving knowledge through meetings, training courses and workshops; and in proving technical support for the elaboration, management and distribution of databases compiled by other divisions.<br>It also provides a Computer Program Service which:<br>• maintains and disseminates comprehensive databases and computer programs;<br>• manages a vast computer program library (with more than 2 500 packages);<br>• distributes thousands of integral data experiments to OECD and to authorised non-OECD countries;<br>• provides courses and workshops on the use of disseminated codes.<br>as well as a Nuclear Data Service (e.g. neutron data libraries) and legacy books (since 2002). |
| Nuclear Science | Recent report on *Research and Test Facilities Required in Nuclear Science and Technology* (NEA, 2009).<br>Compilation and management of the Research and Test Facility DataBase (RTFDB),[29] including records on over 700 nuclear research and test facilities (confirmed with facility operators).<br>Knowledge management:<br>International Reactor Physics Experiments (IRPhE);[30]<br>International Criticality Safety Benchmark Evaluation Project (ICSBEP);<br>International Fuel Performance Experiments (IFPE);<br>Shielding Integral Benchmark and Database (SINBAD). |
| Radioactive Waste Management | In March 2009, a topical session was held on qualified HR in the field of waste management and disposal, considering the extent and health of E&T programmes and plans for HR development and efforts needed to attract young professionals in the fields.<br>Collective opinions: in 1994 – raising initial concern, in 2007 – advocating mechanisms to ensure that knowledge is not lost.<br>Flyer on working in radioactive waste management: www.oecd-nea.org/rwm/documents/rwm-professions-e.pdf. |

28. www.oecd-nea.org/law/isnl/educational_links.htm.

29. www.oecd-nea.org/rtfdb.

30. For the collect of reactor physics experimental data from nuclear facilities worldwide and the provision of qualified benchmark data sets. An IRPhE Handbook is released in DVD format in March every year since 2006.

| Division | Initiative |
|---|---|
| Radiation Protection and Public Health | Periodic surveys on university programmes in radiation protection (in 1996, 2001 and 2005).<br>In May 2009 a meeting topical session was held on "Qualified human resources in the field of radiation protection". |
| Safety | Collective statements (NEA 2008, NEA 2003).<br>Study on the availability and utilisation of facilities supporting safety studies for current and advanced nuclear power reactors (NEA, 2009a).<br>Ongoing activity to develop an understanding of the current needs and activities on Probabilistic Safety Assessment under the auspices of the Working Group on Risk Assessment.<br>Working groups have developed work programmes to deliver E&T through seminars in structural engineering and thermal-hydraulic aspects to young scientists and engineers (e.g. seminars on the transfer of competence, knowledge and experience gained through CSNI activities in the field of thermal-hydraulics, organised every four years since 2004).<br>Continual storing of data from completed joint projects on nuclear safety at the Databank.<br>State-of-the-art reports on various safety issues. |

### *The European Commission*

Within the European Commission three Directorates General (DGs) are, in the main, involved in nuclear matters of education, training or knowledge management; namely: Research and Innovation (DG RTD),[31] Joint Research Centre (DG JRC),[32] and Energy (DG ENER).[33] These directorates have tended to focus on initiatives involving higher education and research institutions, with outputs targeted at regulatory requirements and the supply of high-level expertise. More recently vocational education and consideration of a European Nuclear Skills Passport has been mooted.

The DG RTD has a well defined strategy in the area. Of particular note are the European Nuclear Education Network (ENEN)[34] and the Sustainable Nuclear Energy Technology Platform (SNE-TP).[35]

ENEN was established in 2003 as a non-profit international organisation to preserve and further develop expertise in the nuclear fields through higher education and training. ENEN currently has over 60 members.

SNE-TP was established in 2007. It had a working group in the area of education, training and knowledge management (ETKM WG) which drew on the international infrastructure of ENEN as well as a number of research institutions, major industrial organisations, and a range of trade, skills and learned society bodies.

The DG JRC has an established history of creating, preserving and disseminating nuclear knowledge in research. All DG JRC nuclear research activities are concentrated in the thematic area of nuclear safety and security. Consequently, the education and training activities make use of the synergies between the research sites and are directed towards the needs of stakeholders across industry, research and academia. DG JRC avoids competition with universities by setting up a long cycle of studies of theoretical courses and qualifications which cannot solely be awarded by universities. The DG JRC plan focuses on three areas: 1) nuclear safeguards, security and forensics; 2) nuclear fuel cycle; and 3) basic nuclear science. In the short-, medium- and long-terms these include, respectively:

- establishing a training centre for Safeguards and Nuclear Security;
- establishing programmes of training, seminars, schools and workshops under the three themes;
- establishing a network and facilities for a Euratom School for Nuclear Science.

31. http://ec.europa.eu/research/index.cfm?pg=dg.
32. http://ec.europa.eu/dgs/jrc/index.cfm.
33. http://ec.europa.eu/dgs/energy/index_en.htm.
34. www.enen-assoc.org.
35. www.snetp.eu.

Under the auspices of the DG JRC, the recent launch in 2011 of the European Human Resource Observatory in the nuclear energy sector (EHRO-N)[36] is a move to establish a central information source to optimise the various nuclear initiatives for all nuclear stakeholders in the EU. EHRO-N, was founded in 2009, and is overseen by the JRC Institute for Energy and Transport.[37] The principal objectives of EHRO-N are to maintain a quality-assured database on the short-, medium-, and long-term needs for human resources, to identify gaps and deficiencies in the nuclear E&T infrastructure, and to play an active role in the development of a European scheme of nuclear qualifications and mutual recognition. EHRO-N would communicate regularly relevant data to member states, governments, academic institutions and private organisations, and would also provide recommendations for remedial actions and optimisations to the European Commission.

In 2011, DG JRC also launched the European Nuclear Safety and Security School (EN3S). EN3S is an initiative to reinforce the potential of the expertise and unique facilities housed by the JRC for the purposes of graduate and post-graduate education and training.

The DG ENER launched the European Nuclear Forum (ENEF) in 2007 to explore transparency, opportunities and risks for nuclear energy. This led, not only to EHRO-N (as described above) but also, in 2010, to the founding of ENELA, discussed in Section 2.2.6.

### *Euratom training schemes*

In the EU, the Commission has played and is playing an important role thanks to the Euratom treaty, in supporting research and training on nuclear subjects. It is important that European governments recognise and foster the role of the Commission in supporting HR development.

Euratom,[38] alternatively known as the European Atomic Energy Community, has launched a number of Fission Training Schemes (EFTS) aimed at structuring training and career development across the EU. The ultimate objective of each EFTS is to develop a **European competence passport**.

The 7$^{th}$ Framework Programme (FP-7)[39] of the EU targets research into sustainable energy and security of supply. Five EFTS lie in this area.

**TRASNUSAFE**[40] – aimed at devising two training schemes on nuclear safety culture within a European environment. Based on the evaluation of the specific training needs across Europe the training schemes will include a common generic basis module and four specialised modules that will be validated by means of pilot sessions.

**ENEN III**[41] – training schemes to upgrade knowledge and develop skills, as required by specific positions for nuclear systems suppliers. These comprise four levels: basic nuclear topics for non engineers; design challenges for Generation III NPPs; construction challenges for Generation III NPPs; and design challenges for Generation IV NPPs.

**ENETRAP II**[42] – aimed at developing European high-quality "reference standards" and good practices for education and training in radiation protection, specifically with respect to the radiation protection expert and the radiation protection officer.

**PETRUS II**[43] – Programme for Education, Training and Research on Underground Storage, focusing on the competences required by radioactive waste agencies for professionals working on geological disposal. In this scheme, a Science and Technology Passport is being developed.

36. http://ehron.jrc.ec.europa.eu/.
37. http://iet.jrc.ec.europa.eu/.
38. http://ec.europa.eu/energy/nuclear/euratom/euratom_en.htm.
39. http://cordis.europa.eu/fp7/home_en.html.
40. http://www.enen-assoc.org/en/training/for-nuclear-community/efts-fp7/trasnusafe-fp7.html
41. http://www.enen-assoc.org/en/training/for-nuclear-community/efts-fp7/enen-iii.html
42. http://www.enen-assoc.org/en/training/for-nuclear-community/efts-fp7/enetrap.html
43. http://www.enen-assoc.org/en/training/for-nuclear-community/efts-fp7/petrus.html

**CINCH**[44] – Co-operation in Education in Nuclear Chemistry, focuses on providing a virtual learning platform for collaborative modular postgraduate development.

As illustrated above, the education and training activities of Euratom have traditionally addressed scientists and experts at the higher education level. In recent years, however, attention has turned to training that encompasses the continuous improvement of competencies through borderless mobility and lifelong learning. Therefore, wherever appropriate, the instruments of the European Credit system for Vocational Education and Training are used, in particular the concept of "learning outcomes" and the setting up of "learning agreements". The Euratom training strategy in this area is based on three stages:

- analysis of the needs of society and industry with regard to a common safety culture;
- convergence to a common approach that puts the needs in an EU perspective;
- development of common instruments that meet the needs (ECVET).

### 2.2.6 New emerging trends

*An increasingly global context*

With a small number of technology vendors operating worldwide, the context in which nuclear industry operates is becoming progressively more international (at one point 60 different nationalities were working at Olikuoto-3).

This has spurred the developments of international programmes and initiatives.

Global and regional partnerships committed to enhancing international education and leadership in the peaceful application of nuclear science and technology have been established in the last few years, such as the World Nuclear University (WNU)[45] and the ENELA.[46]

WNU was inaugurated as a non-profit public-private partnership in 2003. It was formed out of a partnership involving industry, academia and governments. The founding partners of WNU are: the global organisations of the nuclear industry (WANO[47] and WNA[48]), the intergovernmental nuclear agencies (IAEA and OECD/NEA), and leading institutions of nuclear learning across 30 countries. WNU activities, designed to address gaps in education and training at the national level by drawing from the wide-ranging strengths of its partners, include:

- Multinational academic co-operation by sharing courses, facilities and students to ensure that the institutions of nuclear learning anticipate the needs of the industry.
- Building nuclear leadership programmes (IAEA, 2007a). Established in 2005 was the internationally peripatetic WNU Summer Institute; an intensive six-week nuclear leadership programme aimed at young (27-37 year-old) nuclear professionals. When fully developed the provision will encompass a summer institute for future leaders, a school of uranium production, an harmonisation forum, executive seminars, regulatory leadership and an advanced nuclear management programme.
- Strengthening of international workforce professionalism.

Originated from an initiative of the ENEF, ENELA was constituted by six nuclear energy companies (AREVA, Axpo AG, EnBW, E.ON Kernkraft GmbH, URENCO Limited and Vattenfall AB) to play a leading role in the European education and training community. It is the ambition of ENELA to train young graduates and high-potential employees from a wide range of academic backgrounds to become future leaders within the European nuclear energy sector. The academy will offer two training programmes. The first one is destined for young graduates from different backgrounds

44. http://cinch-project.eu/
45. www.world-nuclear-university.org/.
46. www.enela.eu.
47. www.wano.info/.
48. www.world-nuclear.org/

(engineering, natural sciences, law, economics, social sciences, etc.) with no professional experience, which will allow them to acquire skills in nuclear management. The second programme will train experienced professionals and senior managers to improve their managerial skills. Finally ENELA will also serve as a think-tank and organise meetings to bring together representatives from the nuclear industry, the political world, the media and civil society. Both courses will provide technical and non-technical training that are mandatory for future middle and top managers.

Individual countries have also increasingly promoted international programmes and transnational collaboration at different levels. In addition to the responsibilities of nations with existing programmes, there is the emerging responsibility of providers, vendor countries (e.g. France and Korea) to form a competent workforce in recipient countries, although the ultimate liability for the implementation of programmes stays with the latter.

In **France,** the French International Nuclear Agency was created in 2008 within the CEA to develop government to government partnerships with countries willing to take advantage of French nuclear competence. In **Korea** KAERI is providing technical support to developing countries, transferring to them its method and programmes for manpower development.

Aspects such as mobility, harmonisation, language use and the need for translation (e.g. in relation to technical manuals and language used by plant operators) have become fundamental issues.

International educational and training programmes are being launched and national courses being open to overseas students (as discussed in Section 2.2.2).

The International Institute for Nuclear Energy (I2EN) was set up in **France** in September 2010 to co-ordinate with academic partners the international recruitment of students, and to promote the French offer for education and training in partner countries. With the support of the training capacities, tools and experience of French nuclear industry, R&D and academic education resources I2EN is also able to create dedicated programmes on demand, for countries choosing bilateral co-operation including assistance in building specific academic capacity as well as internships in France.

International master's degrees in nuclear related subjects, taught in English, have also been recently launched in France:

- Master's Degree in Nuclear Energy Science (MNE).[49]
- Master's Degree in Materials Science for NUclear ENgineering (MANUEN).[50]
- Master's Degree in Sustainable Nuclear Energy and Waste Management (SNEWM).[51]

These are briefly described below.

| Country | Programme | Description | Start date |
|---|---|---|---|
| France | MNE | 2-year international master-level programme by a consortium of engineering schools in the Paris area in conjunction with the University of Paris at Orsay and the INSTN. This programme also receives the support of industrial enterprises (EDF, AREVA, GDF SUEZ) and from CEA. Experimental sessions and training are carried out with EDF simulators. Visits to nuclear sites and a master's theses complement the courses, which are all delivered in English. | September 2009 |
| | MANUEN | 300-hour programme provided by the Grenoble Institute of Technology in close co-operation with EDF and CEA and awarding a degree suitable for both industry and R&D. | 2007 |
| | SNEWM | 2-year programme, in the frame of the *École des Mines de Nantes*, covering reactor physics and operation as well as associated waste management. Numerous other master's degree courses welcome foreign students (about 130 in total for 2009-2010). | September 2010 |

49. www.master-nuclear-energy.fr.
50. http://phelma.grenoble-inp.fr.
51. www.mines-nantes.fr/en/content/view/full/3456.

The process of internationalisation has also allowed the development of wider research opportunities for students, stimulating and attracting them into nuclear and nuclear related R&D. Often aided by the formation of regional and interregional networks such as ENEN and international programmes, considerable progress has also been made in transnational collaboration, with research initiatives acquiring a wider international breath. Transnational collaboration in nuclear research is often a source of favourable "win-win" situations. For instance, despite the presence of research reactors on the national territory, **Korea** has encouraged students to obtain international research experience in **Japanese** facilities, where, conversely, people have been needed to keep the facilities running.

The presence in France of all kinds of nuclear activities and facilities represents a unique opportunity to "train the trainers". Through the collaboration of the major French nuclear players, a new course for trainers, instructors and scholars was launched in 2009. The "train the teachers and instructors" programme has been implemented in close co-operation with interested countries and specifically tailored to their needs and based on an in-depth analysis of the local education system. Broad training, offered in English, includes visits to major French nuclear sites, advanced courses in nuclear engineering, hands-on practice, soft skills such as communication and public acceptance. Internships are also offered. In addition, assistance in designing local training programmes can also be provided.

Some more initiatives are reported below.

| Country | International programmes |
|---|---|
| Belgium | In Belgium, SCK•CEN has instituted its Academy for Nuclear Science and Technology. SCK•CEN's Academy co-ordinates all education and training activities of the Belgian nuclear research centre, and is active on four tracks: *i)* the guidance of young researchers; *ii)* organisation of academic courses in collaboration with Belgian and international universities and organisation of customised training courses for nuclear industry, the medical sector, authorities working in the field of nuclear applications, research, and other sectors such as transport of radioactive materials; *iii)* policy support with regard to E&T matters; and *iv)* research on transdisciplinary aspects of E&T in nuclear.<br>In one university, students spend a year in a foreign nuclear institution as part of their graduate training in nuclear engineering. |
| France | To attract top-quality national and international PhD students and researchers, the INSTN started, in 2007, the "International School on Advanced Studies in Nuclear Engineering". Consisting of nine one-week independent doctoral-level courses taught in English, the school is designed for PhD students but is also open to nuclear-engineering researchers (130 participants attended in 2008-2009). |
| Korea | The nuclear manpower development programme supports a one or two-week visit to a foreign nuclear facility, as well as long-term training programmes of more than six months, for students who achieve outstanding results.<br>Recently, driven by the expectation of increased exports of Korean NPPs, the Ministry of Knowledge and Economy and affiliated organisations have been planning to expand their international co-operation activities and have established the "Nuclear Export Association" to support the government towards enhanced international collaboration. |
| Japan | Under the university, Japanese professors are sent abroad to provide a one-week seminar to students and young researchers in nuclear-developing countries.<br>For provision of technological assistance to developing countries planning to introduce nuclear power, Japan has also launched two international training programmes: the Instructor Training Course (ITC) and the Follow-up Training Course (FTC) under the sponsorship of MEXT. Through these programmes, trainees of participating countries (Bangladesh, Indonesia, Kazakhstan, Malaysia, Philippines, Thailand and Vietnam) are invited from these countries to attend courses in Japan, and experts are sent for training and lecturing activities. |
| Sweden | Since 2008, the Swedish Royal Institute of Technology in Stockholm offers an international MSc in nuclear engineering. The programme has attracted 10-15 students per year. Courses are also open to students participating in other programmes, so that an average attendance of about 25 students per course is reached. |

The process of greater "internationalisation" of nuclear has clearly been reflected also in industry training practices and initiatives: transnational training centres are developed worldwide and international training programmes delivered at domestic and foreign institutes.

 NUCLEAR EDUCATION AND TRAINING: FROM CONCERN TO CAPABILITY, ISBN 978-92-64-17637-9, © OECD 2012

Other examples of industry international training initiatives are given below.

| Country | Transnational training centres |
|---|---|
| France | In partnership with important international academic institutions AREVA has developed training centres worldwide (in France, Germany and the United States). Noteworthy are the large training centre set up in 2009 in Aix-en-Provence, France and the nuclear professional school, founded in co-operation with KIT in Germany. High-level nuclear courses and a combination of compact courses are provided and all teaching methods are used including e-learning, classroom sessions, simulator training and study trips with site tours, and also some specific internships, with practical research work. Worldwide around 500 AREVA courses are currently offered, covering every stage of the fuel cycle, reactor design and construction, and related services, with 100 trainers and several thousand students every year.<br>EDF has also developed a strong internal vocational training organisation for its personnel also offering training worldwide (1.5 million hours per year, with over 650 different operation or maintenance courses). These are supported by a staff of about 700 professionals, including teachers from engineering schools and universities, both in France and abroad. EDF has also strongly promoted the International Masters mentioned above and has developed strategic partnerships with various selected universities and engineering schools.<br>In 2009, a French regional industrial alliance: the Burgundy Nuclear Partnership (BNP)[52] launched the International Nuclear Academy[53] to provide training programmes to upskill, reskill and form HR for businesses in the nuclear sector. The "international nuclear academy" is supported by public fundings. Beside BNP, its partnership extends to institutional and academic bodies and representatives of utility companies and local business. The "international nuclear academy" provides a wide range of training programmes, short seminars and a "Summer University". |
| Korea | In December 2009, KEPCO received approval from the government to launch the KEPCO International Nuclear Graduate School (K-INGS), due to open in March of 2012, the first KEPCO programme completely devoted to nuclear energy. The school will be located next to the Kori NPP, to give easy access for on-the-job training and practical learning experiences. With funding close to KRW 58 billion (USD 49.6 million), K-INGS offers 2-year comprehensive training programmes with specialised courses in nuclear energy planning, operation, and maintenance. These encompass in-house programmes, international co-operation initiatives, such as the "International Nuclear Safety Master Degree Programme" as well as courses for the public and the Nuclear Safety School established in 2004 to form nuclear safety regulators. |

*Mutual recognition, harmonisation and quality assurance*

Enhanced mobility of students and personnel raises issues and aspirations of mutual recognition of qualifications and skills and harmonisation of programmes. Partly linked to increased mobility, is the issue of quality assessment and assurance, which is now becoming more prominent, both in relation to training courses and their outcome and the need for accreditation (including peer review of international training programmes open to external entrants). The ability to ascertain the quality of candidate trainees and students in order to make good selections is also becoming a necessity.

Compatibility amongst different programmes is actively sought, for instance, within the **European Union**. The European Credit Transfer and Accumulation System (ECTS) was introduced in 1999 with the Bologna Declaration and has been adopted by most European universities. Several other programmes (some of which will be discussed later) are sponsored by the European Community in line with such systems. The principal overarching objective is the spreading and sharing a common nuclear safety culture amongst countries with a nuclear programme or wishing to pursue one (including and especially outside the EU). With the same aim, legal and policy bases for training and mobility in Europe have been established, including through the Nuclear Safety Convention and the Nuclear Safety Directive adopted in 2009. This binding directive dictates that: "Member States shall ensure that the national framework in place requires arrangements for education and training to be made by all parties for their staff having responsibilities relating to the nuclear safety of nuclear installations in order to maintain and to further develop expertise and skills in nuclear safety."[54] The Erasmus Mundus programme aims to enhance the quality of higher education and promote dialogue and understanding between people and cultures through mobility and academic co-operation.

---

52. Established in 2005, BNP gathers about 150 businesses from "parent body organisations" such as EDF or AREVA to small and medium enterprises, public laboratories and postgraduate education centres in the region of Burgundy, where a very large activity in design, manufacture and assembly of the primary loop components is concentrated and at the national and international level.

53. www.inuclear-academy.com/.

54. Euratom (2009).

Other prominent initiatives aiming at the standardisation, harmonisation and accreditation of curricula and programmes are listed below.

| Country | Initiative |
|---|---|
| United States | Job Task Analyses (JTAs) leading to training requirement documents know as "INPO ACADs." These proprietary documents form the basis for accredited training in all United States nuclear power plants.<br>Background: following the accident at Three Mile Island the nuclear industry formed the Institute of Nuclear Power Operations (INPO) which subsequently formed the National Academy for Nuclear Training (NANT). Following a Systematic Approach to Training (SAT) NANT established an accredited training system for nuclear workers. INPO maintains the ACAD training documents and the training guidelines based on the JTAs and provides training and support for nuclear power professionals. Accreditation of operator and other technical positions is performed by the independent National Nuclear Accrediting Board.<br>Nuclear Uniform Curriculum Project (NUCP)<br>NUCP is an entry-level technician education programme located at 38 community colleges in partnership with a local nuclear utility. NUCP is run by the Nuclear Energy Institute (NEI) in conjunction with INPO and prepares students for careers in the nuclear energy industry. Its principal goals are to right size the number and type of nuclear technicians for the partner utility. NUCP curricula contains material, mainly knowledge based, that would otherwise be included in the partner utility's training, which is under the requirements laid out in existing INPO ACAD's. Thus when a successful graduate of a NUCP programme is hired, some training can be obviated, shortening the amount of time required for the new plant employee to be fully trained. |
| United Kingdom | Standards and Qualifications Prospectus[55] initiative developed by Cogent, identifying standards and qualifications of relevance to the nuclear industry, families of standard nuclear job roles (Nuclear Job Contexts) to form a detailed job taxonomy.<br>Cogent Technically Higher[56] sets out a roadmap to higher level skills for the science-based industries represented by the Sector Skills Council.<br>National Skills Academy for Nuclear,[57] set out in 2008 to ensure excellence in skills development and provision across the UK nuclear industry, has established a network of High Quality Providers to ensure a delivery of programmes to the highest standards and to develop and implement an industry wide.<br>Nuclear Skills Passport, the passport records nationally recognised skills, competencies and training across the industry across the breadth of the skills pyramid. The Job Contexts are featured on the Skills Passport aligned to the industry agreed training standards, enabling both companies and individuals to carry our detailed training and skills analysis and then plan future skills, training and staffing needs effectively. The Skills Passport will house detailed, current and validated individual learner records enabling and promoting the mobility of staff and the transferability of skills. The industry is making the Skills Passport highly desirable in supply chain tenders so that it can be an effective vehicle for driving up standards across the workforce. Employers have agreed a minimum "bar level" of entry for working in and with the sector which will be recorded and demonstrated on the Skills Passport. The aim of this standard is to ensure that people working in and with the industry understand how and why the nuclear industry is different to other industries and have the right attitudes and behaviours to work safely in this highly regulated industry. |
| France | MESR requires various criteria to validate an education programme. For engineering schools, the *Commission des Titres Ingénieurs* gives an accreditation which is taken into account by the ministry. The new I2EN will release technical analyses to support a label created by CFEN for nuclear education programmes which will complement this organisation. |
| Canada | The master course of engineering offered by several universities within UNENE is accredited by the Ontario Council. |
| Spain | Master courses in several universities have been accredited by the National Accreditation Agency (ANECA), which permits to invite professors from other countries to teach advanced courses. Nuclear education offered by the school of industrial engineers of the Polytechnical University of Madrid has been accredited by ABET for five years. |

### *Innovative methods for education and training*

The spreading of international programmes and networks (see also Section 2.2.1) has often benefitted from improved technological means such as distance learning. Innovative learning methods have been introduced by embracing novel communication systems and means which are well used by the young generation and that, as such, can make education more attractive. The utilisation

55. www.cogent-ssc.com/Publications/Cogent_Qualification_Prospectus_Nuclear.pdf.
56. www.cogent-ssc.com/Higher_level_skills/HE_Strategy.php.
57. www.nuclear.nsacademy.co.uk.

of web-based resources, as well as distance learning, has become a widely adopted practice. This has proved particularly valuable in circumstances where physical or geographical obstacles would prevent the provision of courses or make it significantly more onerous, helping to widely enlarge the pool of prospective students.

In the **United States**, an Internet Reactor Laboratory (IRL)[58] has been established between the nuclear engineering departments at North Carolina State University and at Jordan University of Science and Technology (JUST). The North Carolina State PULSTAR research reactor utilises video conferencing and online reactor instrumentation and data acquisition systems to provide reactor laboratory sessions to students at JUST. This approach can be used at other institutions within or across national borders. To enable the successful implementation of this new modality, in addition to technical aspects, policy and regulatory matters pertaining to issues such as export control had to be addressed.

Within the United States, through distance learning, students can study courses not available at their own university or pursue ones during a semester when they may not be taught (NEA, 2004).

Individual universities, such as the Open University in Madrid, and the Technical University of Catalonia, in co-operation with various organisations (e.g. the **IAEA**) launched in 2010 the "Multimedia on Nuclear Reactor Physics".[59] Several of the educational networks described above provide remote-education platforms. This is the case of:

- JNEN, which uses internet-based systems allowing students to take lectures provided by professors in other universities;
- UNENE, offering distance education for those who would not be able to physically access courses within the Master of Engineering;
- the ANENT (NEA, 2004), through which **Korea**'s well established web-based education and training programmes can be extended to the region.

ENEN has created databases of university courses in Europe,[60] and for the United Kingdom at the portal of the nuclear liaison.[61]

Industry has embraced the use of innovative Internet resources for training and managing knowledge too. In **Canada,** the "CANTEACH" website has been set up as a publicly-accessible repository of all open nuclear information related to education and generated by the industry. It is also used as a resource by UNENE. Some 500 open courses are also provided by KHNP for the industry and the public web-based lectures and training programmes have been developed by the **Korean** KHNP to help remote training. E-learning is used by AREVA in its international training programmes.

### *Craft and technical levels are just as important*

Whilst satisfying the small but important specialist demand for nuclear courses at the higher engineering level is fundamental, adequately addressing the larger demand of craft and technical levels from the sector is just as important, in order to maintain and deploy nuclear programmes robustly anchored on strong safety principles as well as good science and engineering. In the **United States,** industry workforce surveys indicate that there is a growing and persistent need for new technicians to enter the industry, and that, in fact, this dearth in the trades and crafts constitutes the greatest near-term US workforce need, greater than for bachelors or advanced degrees. Vigorous industry initiatives have been initiated in the United States to tackle this challenge, including in the framework of the Nuclear Uniform Curriculum Project (discussed above).

58. www.ne.ncsu.edu/nrp/irl.html.
59. www.xinexus.ch/.
60. www.enen-assoc.org/en/home/database-links.html.
61. www.nuclearliaison.com/nl-courses.

In **Japan**, in 2005 the University of Tokyo has established the Professional School of Nuclear Engineering, which awards qualifications such as "Nuclear Reactor Supervisor" and "Nuclear Fuel Handling Supervisor" as well as the Professional Master Degree. A comprehensive curriculum is taught over one year and a total 16 students per year attend the school, mostly sent by nuclear organisations, such as utilities, nuclear facility manufacturers, as well as regulatory bodies.

In addition to providing more nuclear undergraduate modules, developing new nuclear master level courses, in the **United Kingdom** universities are working with technical colleges, sometimes franchising courses.

In **France**, various specialised curricula have been created, such as the professional "Baccalaureat" for craft, and for technicians, with three types of courses proposed of one, two or three years. These courses lead to the award of specialised diplomas. Most of the graduated are recruited by sub contractors.

However, in general, the supply has not yet reached a sustainable capacity with regard to meeting the demand.

It is important that government support education institutions and young students studying nuclear technology at trade schools or community colleges to ensure there is a well-rounded workforce available for all of the nuclear careers.

*"Nuclearisation" of non-nuclear professionals*

Courses are also being devised for the "nuclearisation" of non-nuclear professionals. In the **United Kingdom** the greatest volume demand is for vocational qualifications and Cogent is working with the industry to develop new courses for specific nuclear skills and is supporting the preparation and roll-out of modular, work-based foundation degrees[62] with the Working Higher Project. The National Skills Academy Nuclear in conjunction with employers and Cogent is developing a Certificate of Nuclear Professionalism. This post-graduate modular certificate, aimed mainly at new graduates, covers managerial, commercial, project management, communication and technical modules which can be delivered flexibly to satisfy the needs of employers.

A new construction skills centre is being erected in West Cumbria to help training employees for jobs on nuclear build projects. Construction work is set to get underway in the spring 2012. It is expected that, upon completion (planned for late 2012) the centre should be able to take on around 280 trainees per year.

In **Sweden** a third-year specialisation in nuclear engineering will be added to an existing three-year bachelor-level mechanics engineering education programme to allow students from any technical college or university with mechanical or electrical engineering to complement their knowledge on nuclear technology. In 2009, Uppsala University has started a nuclear engineering specialisation programme which complements a general engineering programme in energy systems.

The INSTN, in **France**, has increased the offer of seminars and vocational training sessions, including courses in English, some of which in conjunction with ENEN.

### 2.2.7 Conclusions

Since the publication of *Nuclear Education and Training: Cause for Concern?* (NEA, 2000), the general outlook of the nuclear energy industry has changed and many initiatives have been launched to increase E&T capacity.

Challenges still remain, with age profile distributions generally skewed towards high ages and high numbers of impending retirees, strong attrition and, in some countries, the potential deleterious effects and deterrent mechanisms in investments deriving from the situation that may

62. www.cogent-ssc.com/Higher_level_skills/Working_higher.php.

emerge post-Fukushima and from continued economic downturn. In addition, although in some countries student interest in nuclear has turned positive due to more abundant job opportunities and increased environmental understanding of energy needs, in other countries, the trend among young people is to leave technical and scientific disciplines.

There is evidence, however, that progress has been accomplished in addressing certain concerns. Recommendations made in *Cause for Concern* (NEA, 2000) have been heard and stakeholders have taken action.

Improvements have been obtained through transnational programmes as well as the positive engagement of industry.

Industry action has generally been consistent and vigorous, sometimes in conjunction with universities and other parties (e.g. though the establishment of multilateral networks, funding chairs, sponsoring educational programmes, developing and delivering courses, offering internships and, in some cases, opening infrastructure to students). Further, major industrial players have succeeded ramping-up their recruitment rates worldwide.

Since the previous study (NEA, 2000), when the focus was on bridging needs for the existing industry only, with prospects of new build, the context has now changed. In addition to the responsibilities of countries with existing programmes, there is the emerging responsibility of providers and vendor countries to form a competent workforce in recipient countries, although the ultimate liability for the implementation of programmes stays with the latter.

A greater internationalisation has also characterised the nuclear industry, and, linked to it, different questions have arisen, making the discourse in regard to education, training and knowledge management broader and more sophisticated. Aspects such as HR mobility, accreditation, quality control, etc., have emerged as new central topics.

Looking at the pyramid of competence, nuclear professionals at the top remain fundamental and will still be needed in any foreseeable scenario for the safe operation of nuclear installations, the dissemination of knowledge and education and the transmission of safety culture. It has however emerged that there is a growing and persistent need for new technicians to enter the industry, and that, in fact, this dearth in the trades and crafts sometimes constitutes the greatest near-term workforce need (e.g. in the **United Kingdom** and the **United States**). Adequately addressing the larger demand of craft and technical levels from the sector is paramount to maintaining and deploying nuclear programmes robustly anchored on strong safety principles. Some actions have already been reported in this respect (e.g. in the way of inter-university consortia and college partnerships with universities, which, sometime have also franchised courses) but more needs to be done, as further discussed in Chapter 3.

The integration of national academic and research institutes within international frameworks has generally grown. It is widely recognised that a strong and increased participation in international research programmes and the greater involvement of industry in research and training must be pursued and can considerably improve the situation, in certain countries (e.g. in **Spain**).

While other stakeholders have acted, without government participation, there is generally limited ability to change the educational system.

In many countries governments have commissioned manpower assessments (e.g. Finland, France, Japan, the United Kingdom, the United States, etc.), often through ad hoc councils and bodies established for the purpose of labour market research and workforce development. Active monitoring of demand and supply capacity is an important step for HRD; but, in order for it to bear effective and long-lasting benefits, it should be conducted on an ongoing basis, with assessments undertaken regularly and frequently for systematic planning.

The results of recent manpower assessments have, in a few cases, triggered government actions to address emerging gaps. In some instances governments have provided specific support to university programmes and research, which has contributed, in a few countries, to reversing the declining trends of subscription in nuclear engineering. Noteworthy are the cases of France, Sweden, the United Kingdom and the United States.

However, across the board, governments have not acted strategically and coherently. Governments are also responsible for instating favourable conditions; contradictory and shifting energy policies have a negative effect on student interest in nuclear-related disciplines.

HRD long-term planning still remains key, while systematic approaches to achieve competency still appear to be somewhat deficient.

## 2.3 Present use of research infrastructure for education and training in NEA member countries

### 2.3.1 *Introduction*

Research reactors (RR), critical assemblies (CA) and thermal-hydraulic facilities (THF) can have multiple usages. Indeed, they can be used to carry out research, provide services and contribute to education and/or teaching, including the preparation of theses and dissertations. The effective use of a research facility for E&T purposes depends however on financial and organisational factors. As no comprehensive quantitative information on such use has been reported yet for NEA member countries a survey was performed within the framework of the present study [comprehensive databases on world RRs exist, notably IAEA Research Reactors Database (RRDB)[63] and the International Group on RRs (IGORR)[64] database; these, however do not report quantitative information on the E&T use of such facilities for purposes]. Building on a recent activity developed within the EU Sustainable Nuclear Energy Technology Platform (SNE-TP, 2010), the survey measures the availability and level of use of nuclear research infrastructure for E&T. Owners or operators of facilities were requested to provide information by means of a questionnaire (reproduced in Appendix 3). The present section reports the outcomes of this investigation, whereas some numerical data are summarised in Appendix 3. It should be noted that no attempt has been made to analyse availability and needs for the broader use of research infrastructure for nuclear science and technology, or to provide a comprehensive assessment on the status of ageing of research facilities. Such aspects have been thoroughly analysed in a recent OECD/NEA report: *Research and Test Facilities Required in Nuclear Science and Technology* (NEA, 2009), which also led to the compilation of the Research and Test Facility Database (RTFDB),[65] containing information on over 700 nuclear test and research facilities (not limited to NEA member countries). It is the intent of this ad hoc expert group to incorporate the newly gathered information on E&T uses of facilities in the RTFDB. The Committee on the Safety of Nuclear Installations (CSNI) has also recently published the SFEAR report on safety issues, research needs and supporting research facilities associated with water reactors in NEA member countries (NEA, 2009a).

Section 2.3.2 examines the use of RRs and CAs for different geographical regions, while the contribution of various categories of THFs to E&T is analysed in Section 2.2.3 (both for the period 2005-2009). In both areas, it is shown that much more could be done with the existing equipment for the benefit of education and training. It also appears that new equipment is required to replace ageing facilities.

Although computer simulations and full scale simulators today enable the delivery of many training exercises focussing on practical problems of reactor physics, plant operation, safety and thermal-hydraulics, there are strong arguments to justify that software simulations alone cannot provide the full range of practice required for a complete trainee preparation. Indeed, there remains a need for the student/trainee to experience work environment conditions which are closer to the real world, with radiological protection implications, dealing with pipes and vessels under pressure and at high temperatures, measuring instruments, etc. Moreover, practical training in real laboratories provides an initiation to nuclear safety culture through the organisational and technical issues involved.

63. http://nucleus.iaea.org/RRDB/RR/ReactorSearch.aspx.
64. www.igorr.com/scripts/home/publigen/content/templates/show.asp?P=785&L=EN&ITEMID=6.
65. www.oecd-nea.org/rtfdb/.

In Section 2.2.4, some recommendations are formulated for a more intensive use of the nuclear research infrastructure surveyed.

### *2.3.2 The present use of research reactors and critical assemblies*

*North America*

The case of **Canada** illustrates the typical situation. Several RRs were identified as being used for E&T; this is the case for almost all of the SLOWPOKE type reactors. However, in general, such facilities are far from being exploited to their full potential for E&T. The following examples show that an increased use is possible. In Ontario, facilities located at the Royal Military College of Canada and those run by the McMaster University appear to be very actively used for education purposes, but yet it is reported that a substantial increase could be feasible (from 200 to 300 and from 175 to 350 students per year respectively). At AECL, Chalk River Laboratories, the Zed-2 facility, which celebrated its $50^{th}$ anniversary in 2010, is not currently used for E&T. However, its management suggests that it "could be used as a hands-on reactor physics laboratory by undergraduate and graduate students and by nuclear industry professionals. Up to three graduate students could be accommodated at any given time. Requirements would depend on the programme(s) set up for the students, and funding for the students from outside AECL would be required."

A recent restructuring within the nuclear industry in Canada may also improve educational initiatives. The commercial arm of AECL at Sheridan Park, Mississauga, including its CANDU reactor line, has been sold to SNC Lavalin and will become CANDU Energy Inc. The AECL research arm, mainly at Chalk River Laboratories, will in effect become more of a national nuclear laboratory, with a broadened mandate. This mandate is still under development, but is expected to include much more co-operation with universities, including making CRL facilities more available to university students and researchers, hosting students on-site as part of their degree work, etc.

In the **United States**, there are 32 universities nuclear engineering, nuclear technology and health-physics degree programmes accredited by ABET (ABET, 2012). Most, but not all of these programmes are at universities with a research reactors. These reactors are used to some extent in the educational courses at their universities and other schools with which they may have reactor sharing programmes. Typically there is a nuclear measurements laboratory or reactor operations course that utilises the reactor for some demonstrations and experiments. Some students get trained and pass a federal operator's examination to become licensed reactor operators. Also, some of the students who earned graduate degrees will have utilised the reactor on their campus for performing their research, but the majority have made use of other facilities. The reactors are used by other researchers in such fields as geology or material science and by industrial users for various purposes such as radiography or to measure the effects of exposure on their products. It is fair to say that there is an opportunity for more educational utilisation at most facilities.

All university research reactors receive support from the federal government in terms of fuel and most have received infrastructure grants for such projects as upgrading reactor instrumentation and making other improvements to enhance utilisation for researchers and other users. The facilities are generally in fairly good shape. Suggestions for better use of the existing facilities for doing more education and training most commonly would be in having staff dedicated to that function.

Use of the university reactors for training operators at commercial reactors is not typically done since all power reactors have large full scale reactor simulators. However, some utilities use RRs to enhance training of reactor fundamentals such as reactivity feedback and basic reactor control for engineers and other plant workers.

### *Asia*

The survey results suggest that in **Japan**, where 6 out of 14 RRs include E&T activities, the number of students accommodated could almost double (see Table A3.1 in Appendix 3). A major shutdown was also reported: that of the reactor at the University of Tokyo (YAYOI). Noteworthy are the efforts at the Kyoto University, Reactor Research Institute (KURRI) where a joint reactor laboratory course at graduate level has been offered every summer since 1975 by nine associated Japanese universities. Using the Kyoto University Critical Assembly (KUCA), on average 4 doctoral theses and 4 master theses are prepared each year, while 200 hours of practical teaching are organised for 150 students.

**Korea** has only one RR, called high-flux advanced neutron application reactor (HANARO), which in Korean language, means "uniqueness". Its use for education, with 240 hours of lab sessions for about 300 students, seems to match the local needs.

### *Australia*

OPAL, commissioned in 2006, is an open pool advanced multi-purpose LWR reactor, designed to fulfil commercial and research activities (Storr, 2010). Apart from training internal staff and supporting PhD theses, it could be used to facilitate broader training within the field of nuclear engineering. Students, trainers and international workshops relating to nuclear reactor engineering could benefit from the use of the facility. Training rooms and facilities, including a reactor simulator, are currently available and are used for the training of reactor personnel. However, funding would be required to provide external training, which would need to be scheduled to fit with the overall utilisation requirements of the reactor.

### *Europe*

(See also SNE-TP, 2010) In Europe, four groups of countries can be distinguished:

- A first group includes those countries which do not operate power reactors or research reactors and have minimal needs to educate competent people in nuclear engineering. These are: Denmark, Estonia, Ireland, Latvia, Luxemburg and Malta.
- A second group represents those countries, like Bulgaria,[66] Lithuania, the Slovak Republic, Spain and Sweden, which currently operate power reactors but not research reactors. These countries, therefore, rely on training facilities abroad or on simulators for practical training.
- A third group includes those countries: Austria, Greece, Italy, Norway, Poland and Portugal, which do not operate power reactors but run one or several RRs. The survey shows that for all countries of this group but Norway and Poland, E&T is offered in RRs operated locally.
- Countries of the fourth group have both power and research reactors.

Roughly one half of the RRs are used for education at MSc/BSc levels: 28 out of 60 in countries within EU27+. Only a few are really dedicated to civilian training. Taking the arbitrary criterion of 120 hours of operation for didactical purposes, only the 8 reactors listed below exceed this level, and at least three of these are due to shut down in the next 5 to 10 years: AKR-2 (D), CONSORT (UK),[67] CROCUS (CH), ISIS (F),[68] SUR-ULM (D), Training Reactor (H),[69] TRIGA II (A),[70] VR1 (CZ), and, hopefully in the future, IRT (BLG) within the NuTEC structure.

Such limited use of RRs for practical training can be explained as follows:

- Running lab sessions is only possible on small RRs; bigger facilities are too expensive or inappropriate for teaching purposes.

66. It should be noted that Bulgaria has a research reactor: the IRT-Sofia, which however, is presently shut down for major refurbishment and conversion into a low power reactor.

67. Anticipated shutdown within the next two to five years.

68. Anticipated shutdown in 2015.

69. Anticipated shutdown in 2026.

70. Anticipated shutdown in 2020.

- Universities are committed to offer lab sessions to the students, while, in general, education does not figure strongly in the mission and purposes of research centres. However, running experimental facilities and a fortiori a research reactor in a university has become very difficult due to the financial burden, including costs for the enforcement of more stringent safety and security regulations.
- Although no investigation on the demand side has been completed within this study, it can be inferred that, due to the relatively small number of students registered in nuclear engineering programmes, at the present time there is adequate correspondence between the offer and the demand for laboratory sessions. This emerged for the EU countries in the EU SNE-TP study where the demand was also assessed (SNE-TP, 2010).
- No urgent need to increase the supply capacity has hence been detected.
- Not all academics are convinced that hands-on training is a mandatory part of nuclear engineering education (see also SNE-TP, 2010). Sometime computer simulation is deemed more beneficial.[71]

It is also noted that in EU27+ the numbers of PhD and MSc theses conducted in RRs are quite similar, approximately 75 per year each. It is difficult to develop experimental research on a reactor within a period limited only to one academic year; this may explain why the number of MSc theses is limited and comparable to those for doctoral research. However, the situation is not the same in Japan where the ratio between the numbers of MSc and PhD theses is of the order of 3.

The survey has shown that there is a substantial potential for increase in the number of students that could be accommodated: at least by 40% and possibly much more if the numbers of technicians and supervisors were increased accordingly in the facilities.

### *2.3.3 The present use of thermal-hydraulic facilities*

A wide variety of THF exists around the world, each facility having its own objectives, with not much duplication. A brief review is provided in this section, where THF facilities are categorised according to their size and use. Contrary to RRs, THFs are not so susceptible to ageing and new facilities are regularly built. Reliable data on their use for E&T are difficult to collect, due to their vast number and great diversity. Nevertheless the survey has clearly shown that the potential for increasing the number of students is much higher than for reactors. According to the information received from a number of facility operators, an increase of students by a factor of 3 would seem feasible. Finally, as observed for RRs, the number of doctoral theses and that of master theses developed in THF facilities are similar. However, compared to those conducted in RRs, numbers are much lower; in Europe (EU+), for instance, PhD theses are about 20 per year, like MSc theses, i.e. about one third of those conducted in RRs.

#### *Very large and complex THFs – Integral test facilities*

Some very large and complex THFs were built in the 1970s in order to support safety studies for different types of LWRs and validate safety codes. Some of them have been dismantled (e.g. **LOBI** at JCR-Ispra in Italy and **BETSY** in France). Some others are still in use or have been built more recently. A few examples are considered below.

Operated within the ROSA programme, **LSTF**, in Japan, reproduces a typical full pressure and full height 4-loops PWR. Another example is **THYNC**, a test section that simulates parallel core channels of BWR in combination with its attached mother loop inherited from CCTF: PWR 2D3D refill-reflood large-scale facility. The mother loop can provide steam-water two-phase flow at PWR nominal operating conditions into the test section that can be replaced according to the research objectives. If necessary, both facilities LSTF and THYNC could be used for E&T, but the cost would be very high.

71. In Europe some students graduate in nuclear engineering without having seen a reactor at work. Too many sources of funding are spent for computational and theoretical work while experimental work is not always favoured especially at universities (SNE-TP, 2010).

In Korea, **ATLAS**, the Advanced Thermal-Hydraulic Test Loop for Accident Simulation, is an example of a more recently built large-scale thermal-hydraulic integral effect test facility, to study evolutionary pressurised water reactors. Whilst it is reported that, with the implementation of sophisticated instruments, it could be made available for education use at doctoral level, presently this facility is not used for E&T purposes.

At the Rossendorf Research Centre in Germany two test facilities are operated: **TOPFLOW**, which was designed to investigate stationary and transient phenomena in two-phase flow with the purpose of developing and validating models used in computational fluid dynamics codes, and **ROCOM**, which was erected for the investigation of coolant mixing in a PWR pressure vessel. These are not used for E&T except for a few students preparing theses.

This is also the case for the test facility **PANDA**, in Switzerland, originally designed and used for investigating integral containment system behaviour, in particular for advanced passive (Generation III+) BWRs. Currently, the facility is being used for basic containment thermal-hydraulics studies, e.g. in relation to the hydrogen problem

More extensive use for E&T is pursued in the two following THFs: **SPES** in Italy, an experimental facility equipped to simulate and study the behaviour of a nuclear power plant both during operational and accidental transients, and, in Hungary, **PMK-2**, a scaled-down model of the Paks nuclear power plant equipped with VVER-440/213-type reactors of Soviet design.

Finally, in Finland, **PACTEL** is a unique example of an out-of pile integral facility operated by a university (the Lappeenranta University of Technology). This facility is currently used for E&T purposes, with PhD and MSc theses as well as laboratory sessions.

As for France, although several sets of experimental facilities, grouped in platforms, are run for research, their use for education is limited to the preparation of theses.

*Heavy liquid metal facilities*

A second category of THFs consists of facilities dedicated to studies on flow and heat transfer phenomena involving liquid metals (sodium, lead, lead-bismuth eutectic, etc.). These are related to Generation IV projects and include the development of new components and instrumentation. Participation of students is limited to theses, but one should not underestimate the importance of these facilities for the future, in particular to train technicians in the practical aspects of liquid metal utilisation. It is noteworthy to remember the training delivered for many years in this field at the "School of sodium" at CEA/Cadarache (France).

*Facilities devoted to the analysis of severe accidents*

A number of facilities are devoted to aspects related to severe accidents: core disassembly, steam explosion, molten fuel flow and cooling, hydrogen releases and explosions, aerosols, decontamination of gaseous systems by sprays, autocatalytic recombiners, particle beds (debris) dryout, concrete-corium interaction, etc. Such topics can form the subject of theses.

*Experiments with down-scaled loops and/or with simulant fluids, or analytical experiments*

The most common THFs of this type consist of loops down-scaled in terms of size, pressure or flow rate, in test facilities operated with simulant fluids such as air-water, freons, helium (instead of hydrogen), and/or facilities for analytical or fundamental studies. Research on these THFs focuses on:

- Heat transfer and fluid flow phenomena like critical heat flux (CHF), post-CHF and re-flood heat transfer, natural circulation, pebble beds, boron mixing, etc.
- Performance of components, such as T-junctions, valves, safety depressurisation and venting systems, downcomer boiling, rod bundle thermal-hydraulics, CANDU Header, BWR condensation pool, passive cooling systems, etc.

The use of these loops for E&T is very variable from case to case.

*Loops with a test section inserted in a research reactor*

A last category includes the in-pile loops. Examples are the high temperature helium loop (HTHL) and super critical water loop (SCWL) at NRI-Řež (Czech Republic). These two test sections are not used for education, although they could be made available for doctoral research. This is generally the case for such facilities, which are normally not accessible for E&T, except for a small number of PhD theses.

### 2.3.4 Advocating a more intensive use of nuclear research infrastructure for E&T

The ad hoc expert group recognises the benefits of a more intensive use of nuclear research infrastructure for laboratory sessions. Full advantage should be taken of existing facilities, including amenable industry research infrastructure. Computer models and computer simulations do not replace laboratory sessions but should enhance their use. Indeed, through hands-on training, trainees are confronted with hard technology, especially if they have to develop solutions in a nuclear environment with radiological constraints. Of course, linked computer simulations bring the added benefit of an increased degree of understanding and theoretical extrapolation, but they cannot replace hands-on experience, especially given the continued emphasis needed on safety culture.

The involvement of PhD students in research programmes using RRs and THFs is a usual way to improve the depth of research and to prepare the take-over by well-trained and educated people. This involvement could be further extended, and therefore efforts should be made towards the financial support of non proprietary research. The involvement of students in MSc theses is also commendable within the limits imposed by the time constraints for both the theses and the research projects.

In the framework of rapidly growing student mobility, information on the topics offered for experimental theses as well as grant availability should be made more easily accessible to attract good students from all over the world. Regional nuclear engineering education networks like ANENT and ENEN could play a role in facilitating the spread of this type of information, whilst industry should offer financial support in the form of grants and placements for internships. "Experimental weeks" could also be organised by these university networks to ease the practical organisation of laboratory sessions.

NEA (2004) testified to the deterioration of the financial situation of research institutes, in many countries due to cuts in public funding and to tough competition in the niche market where they sell their services and products. Although this outlook seems to have changed in some countries, with funds being directed to R&D and the support of research infrastructures e.g. in United States (with the allocation of substantial funding from DOE) and in Belgium (where the government contributes financially to the MYRRHA project), warnings have been raised (NEA, 2009 and 2009a) over the fact that many expensive and unique facilities are due to close over the next few years (NEA, 2009). Many RRs were put into operation in the 1960s and are thus clearly ageing. Some of them have already shut down and a substantial number is awaiting the same fate. As an example, 245 reactors were reported as operating in 2007 (IAEA, 2007b) two thirds of which were older than 30 years, while 272 research reactors were operating in 2004 (IAEA, 2003). Within the European member states of the OECD, R2 – a 50 MW(th) reactor in Sweden – was shut down in 2005 (Studsvik NEWS, 2005). In France OSIRIS, a 70 MW(th) reactor which has been in operation since 1966, is expected to shut down in 2015 and Phénix was shut down in 2010. Many other RRs are reported to have commenced operation within the same 1950-1960s time frame and they continue to operate today within current and individual licensing periods of up to about 10 years.

## References

ABET (2012), List of accredited Nuclear Engineering, Nuclear Engineering Technology and Health Physics programs. www.abet.org. March 2012.

CEWD (2008), *Gaps in the Energy Workforce Pipeline: 2008 CEWD Survey Results, 2008*, Center for Energy Workforce Development. www.cewd.org/documents/CEWD_08Results.pdf.

CNHRD (2010), *Report of the Council of Nuclear HRD*, Council on Nuclear Human Resources Development, Tokyo, Japan (in Japanese).

Commonwealth of Australia (2006), *Uranium Mining, Processing and Nuclear Energy – Opportunities for Australia?*, Report to the Prime Minister, Department of the Prime Minister and Cabinet, Australia.

DOE (2010), *Nuclear Energy Research and Development Roadmap, Report to Congress*, US Department of Energy, April 2010, Washington DC, United States, Available at http://nuclear.gov/pdfFiles/NuclearEnergy_Roadmap_Final.pdf.

EC (2009), *Nuclear Safety in a Situation of Fading Nuclear Experience*, European Commission, Brussels, Belgium.

Euratom (2009), *Establishing a Community framework for the nuclear safety of nuclear installations*, Article 7, Council Directive 2009/71/EURATOM of 25 June 2009, Available on http://eur-lex.europa.eu/LexUriServ/LexUriServ.do?uri=OJ:L:2009:172:0018:0022:EN:PDF.

IAEA (2003), *International Conference on Research Reactors Utilization, Safety, Decommissioning, Fuel and Waste Management website*, 10-14 November 2003, Santiago, Chile, Organised by the IAEA.

IAEA (2006), *Competency Assessments for Nuclear Industry Personnel*, IAEA, Vienna, Austria. Available at www-pub.iaea.org/MTCD/publications/PDF/Pub1236_web.pdf

IAEA (2007), *Milestones in the Development of a National Infrastructure for Nuclear Power*, IAEA, Vienna, Austria. Available at www-pub.iaea.org/MTCD/publications/PDF/Pub1305_web.pdf.

IAEA (2007a), *The World Nuclear University: New Partnership in Nuclear Education*, IAEA, Vienna, Austria. Available at www-pub.iaea.org/MTCD/Publications/PDF/IAEA-WNU_web.pdf.

IAEA (2007b), *International Conference on Research Reactors: Safe Management and Effective Utilization website*, 5-9 November 2007, Sydney, Australia, Organised by the IAEA.

IAEA (2009), *Development of Knowledge Portals for Nuclear Power Plants*, IAEA, Vienna, Austria. Available at www.iaea.org/inisnkm/nkm/documents/Pub1377_web.pdf

IAEA (2009a), *Managing Human Resources in the Field of Nuclear Energy*, IAEA, Vienna, Austria. Available at www-pub.iaea.org/MTCD/publications/PDF/Pub1397_web.pdf

IAEA (2010), *International Conference on Human Resource Development for Introducing and Expanding Nuclear Power Programmes*, 14-18 March 2010, Abu-Dhabi, United Arab Emirates, Organised by IAEA www-pub.iaea.org/MTCD/Meetings/Announcements.asp?ConfID=38090.

IAEA (2010a), *Educational Programme in Nuclear Security*, IAEA, Vienna, Austria. Available at www-pub.iaea.org/MTCD/publications/PDF/Pub1439_web.pdf

IAEA (2011), *Status and Trends in Nuclear Education*, IAEA, Vienna, Austria. Available at www-pub.iaea.org/MTCD/publications/PDF/P1475_web.pdf.

IAEA (2011a), *Workforce Planning for New Nuclear Power Programmes*, IAEA, Vienna, Austria. Available at www-pub.iaea.org/MTCD/Publications/PDF/Pub1477_web.pdf

Khan, R., Böck, H. and M. Villa (2008), *Management of Nuclear Knowledge*.

KSU (2009), *Operating Experience from Swedish Nuclear Power Plants*, Available at Kärnkraftsäkerhet och Utbildning AB, KSU, Studsvik, Sweden, http://www.ksu.se/wp-content/uploads/2011/05/Arsrapport2009_eng1.pdf

 NUCLEAR EDUCATION AND TRAINING: FROM CONCERN TO CAPABILITY, ISBN 978-92-64-17637-9, © OECD 2012

NEA (2000), *Nuclear Education and Training: Cause for Concern?*, OECD, Paris, France.

NEA (2003), *Collective Statement Concerning Nuclear Safety Research – Good Practice and Closure Criteria*, OECD, Paris, France.

NEA (2004), *Nuclear Competence Building*, OECD, Paris, France.

NEA (2007), Proposed Statement by the NEA Steering Committee for Nuclear Energy regarding a Government Role in Ensuring Qualified Human Resources in the Nuclear Field, NEA/NE(2007)9, September 2007, OECD, Paris, France.

NEA (2008), *CSNI Collective Statement on Support Facilities for Existing and Advanced Reactors*, OECD, Paris, France.

NEA (2009), *Research and Test Facilities Required in Nuclear Science and Technology*, OECD, Paris, France.

NEA (2009a), *Support and Test Facilities for Existing and Advanced Reactors* (SFEAR), Report of the Senior Group of Experts on Nuclear Safety Research (SESAR), OECD, Paris, France.

NESTet (2011), *Nuclear Engineering Science and Technology*, Education and Training Conference, 15-18 May 2011, Prague, Organised by the European Nuclear Society.

SNE-TP (2010), *Current and Future Uses of Nuclear Infrastructure in Europe*, SNE-TP – Working Group ETKM – Subgroup 4.

SDC (2006), *The Role of Nuclear Power in a Low Carbon Economy*, Sustainable Development Commission, London, United Kingdom. Available at www.sd-commission.org.uk/data/files/publications/SDC-NuclearPosition-2006.pdf.

Storr G. (2010), Private communication from Greg Storr, Australian Nuclear Science and Technology Organisation (ANSTO).

Studsvik NEWS (2005), *Hot Spring for R2 but Now an Era is Over*, Studsvik NEWS, June.

WNN (2011), *New Reactors, New Workforce*. Available at www.world-nuclear-news.org/NN_New_reactors_new_workforce_0112111.html.

*Chapter 3*

# Towards a blueprint for workforce development

## 3.1 The benefits of a competent nuclear workforce

Prior to this study, *Cause for Concern* in 2000 and many reports on skills for nuclear power published since have focused, appropriately, either on the high end of the skills spectrum or on supply issues predicated on the capability of education and research establishments (e.g. IAEA, 2011; EC, 2009; SNE-TP, 2010). While these skills are critical to the industry, and nuclear specialist supply comes mainly from such routes, **the industry employs, by a large margin, many more non-nuclear specialists (e.g. mechanical, electrical, civil, instrumentation and control), as well as technical and craft personnel, than nuclear specialists**. Further, induced employment in a growing contractor supply chain extends the scope required for training and development for competence.

In the nuclear industry ensuring a competent workforce is paramount for the safe operation of any nuclear-related activity, and in instilling the confidence of stakeholders. National and international policies and regulations apply to this industry. These require the highest specifications of safety and reliability in both the technology and in the competence of those employed to design, build, operate, maintain and decommission nuclear facilities. Independent non-governmental bodies support and advise here. Undoubtedly, for employees working on a nuclear licensed site or in the supply chain of a nuclear operator, safe behaviours are critical, particularly with increased proximity to the "nuclear island" and controlled areas. The preponderance of human factors at all stages and levels is notable. This has been further emphasised by the impact of human factors in incidents and accidents, highlighting the importance of safety culture and safety training in nuclear operations.

Taking a high-level view, governments use regulators to ensure utility companies are licensed to operate nuclear reactors safely and that vendors design, supply and build safely. Under these circumstances, both the utilities and the vendors rely on verifiable levels of competence in the workforce. This is required not only for their own workforces but also for those in the supply chain from whom products and services are contracted, and for whose competence they may ultimately be held responsible. A framework for competent workforce training and education at all levels could lead the way to comparability and possibly interoperability of standards for training and qualifications, enabling mobility and retention of suitably qualified and experienced personnel and better confidence in the safe and secure deployment of nuclear technology. It may also provide a robust basis for international labour market research, scenario planning and human resource observatories, supporting those initiatives to develop "passports" or licences to practise for competence assurance and acting as guidance for the safe and secure development of nuclear personnel in developing countries. The overarching goal of such an effort is to create an efficacious system for training and education leading to competent workers imbued with adequate knowledge, skills and a "safety culture" attitude.

However, national diversity in regulatory practice and approaches to the supply, demand and accreditation of education and training means that there are, to date, no internationally accredited frameworks for competence assurance. This is not to say that competence frameworks do not exist at different levels; rather, that there is a broad resource of accredited good practice that could be built into a coherent framework of international reference.

A process to develop a taxonomy, or classification system, for nuclear job roles is presented herein, that draws on elements of various such systems in several countries and provides an outline for a set of typical jobs in the nuclear industry.

Information has been contributed by different countries and for consistency in capturing national information, a template was issued to all contributing organisations. Each contributor was asked to provide a limited number of representative but detailed case inputs. To bring the data into alignment a "normalisation" was applied to template returns to account for variations in terminology, style and culture.

The resulting system is of course nominal; it is not exhaustive or final (neither in depth nor in spread), nor does it provide a unique taxonomy solution. Alternative taxonomies may be devised to better represent or analyse particular characteristics, using different approaches to address different needs. Two examples of studies adopting job taxonomies are reported in Appendix 5, which, to some extent demonstrate this.

Building on commonalities this framework taxonomy establishes an initial platform, upon which individual countries and organisations can overlay their own specific requirements, providing an indication of how alternative and more comprehensive classifications may be more fully developed.

## 3.2 Classifying competence

A job taxonomy is an in-depth skills classification system which allows the mapping and characterisation of discrete job profiles according to the specific tasks, the responsibilities and activities the role entails, the competencies needed to fulfil them, as well as the associated entry level qualification, training and experience requirements.

Definitions which this framework taxonomy relies upon include: scope, sector, function, job roles, occupational level, competence and competency. These are captured in the ensuing text.

### *3.2.1 Scope*

The scope of the proposed framework taxonomy is bounded by the lifecycle of a nuclear reactor, i.e. new build, operation and decommissioning, but includes the closely related areas of research reactors, and nuclear regulation (covered in the present study to a lesser degree of detail). It is noted that the nuclear fuel cycle is wider than this and that the scope of this approach thereby excludes areas such as ore mining, uranium extraction and enrichment, fuel processing and reprocessing. The reason for limiting the scope is that only a few countries either have or are likely to deploy full capability across the entire nuclear fuel cycle, yet most established and aspiring civil nuclear nations would require at minimum the identified fields of new build, regulation, operation and decommissioning.

It must be stressed that this taxonomy neither recognises any specific reactor technology dependence (e.g. reactor type: pressurised water, boiling water, gas-cooled, etc.), nor does it hold within scope all aspects of conventional engineering such as structural steelwork, concreting or mechanical installation, unless nuclear codes or components are involved. Similarly, clerical roles such as accounting, personnel management, legal, commercial, etc., are excluded, except for those roles requiring knowledge of training and nuclear specialisation that would apply to the selection of personnel or the training of personnel. In this way the taxonomy stays close to the degree of nuclearisation required of the workforce.

### *3.2.2 An illustrative taxonomy – Classification hierarchy*

Within its defined *scope*, the framework taxonomy adopts a hierarchical approach, categorising job roles first by *sector* and secondly by *function*. Within each function of each sector, job roles are specified with key competencies at the various occupational levels.

**Figure 3.1: An illustrative taxonomy – classification hierarchy**

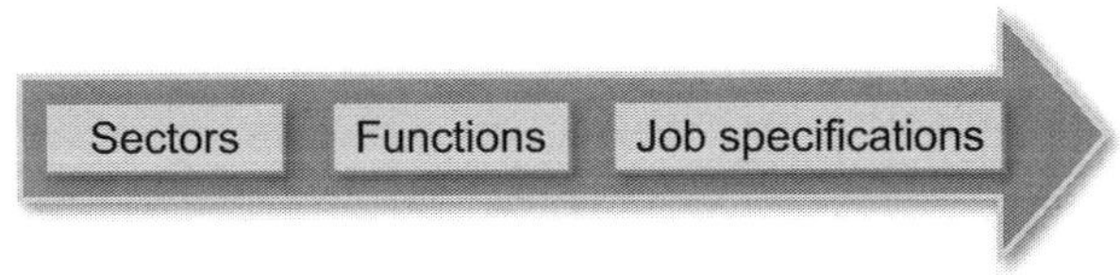


For illustration, the taxonomy hierarchy (sectors, functions and job specifications) (Figure 3.1) adopted is described in some detail for the workforce in nuclear power plants, in research reactors and the regulator respectively in Sections 3.2.3, 3.2.4 and 3.2.5.

*Sectors and functions*

**Figure 3.2: An illustrative taxonomy – sectors and functions**

| Sectors | Functions |
|---|---|
| **Nuclear power plant** New build | • Design<br>• Supply<br>• Construction<br>• Commission |
| **Nuclear power plant** Operation | • Operation<br>• Maintenance<br>• Waste management<br>• Safety and environment |
| **Nuclear power plant** Decommissioning | • Decommissioning operation<br>• Maintenance<br>• Waste management<br>• Safety and environment |
| **Nuclear research reactors** | • Design and engineering<br>• Utilisation<br>• Operation and control |
| **Nuclear regulation** | • Assessment and review<br>• Authorisation<br>• Inspection and enforcement<br>• Regulation and guidance |

Sectors are defined by the taxonomy according to the objective for which the workforce is employed, for example, in the nuclear power plant taxonomy, new build, operation, decommissioning and regulation (Figure 3.2).

Functions are defined by the taxonomy according to the phases or segregated activities within which specific job roles are deployed; for instance maintenance, waste management, safety and environment, operation and control.

Each of the functions includes many job roles with demonstrable nuclear and non-nuclear activities. A number of exemplar job roles that typify each sector and function have been selected for illustration and are listed in Appendix 4.

### *Job role specifications*

The taxonomy adds a job specification layer for each function of each sector. This defines the greatest level of detail in the process, with specifications of occupational levels and competencies required, as well as sets of initial qualifications,[1] advisory training and continuous professional development to support them, as depicted in Figure 3.3.

**Figure 3.3: An illustrative taxonomy – job specifications**

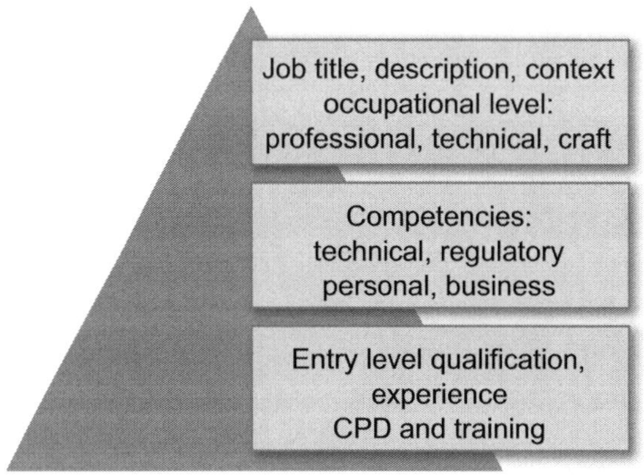

Job title, description, context
occupational level:
professional, technical, craft
Competencies:
technical, regulatory
personal, business
Entry level qualification,
experience
CPD and training


Tables A4.5-A4.8 in Appendix 4 list 30 job specifications across the sectors and functions of the taxonomy. The job roles selected for detailed characterisation in each case are deemed as representative and important to the sectors and functions. These are neither comprehensive nor fully developed, but are provided as information advice and guidance on nuclear workforce development.

The key occupational categories of "professional", "technical" and "craft" have been used. These accord, to a large degree, with the International Standard Classification of Occupations (ISCO), which is an International Labour Organisation (ILO) classification structure and is part of the international family of economic and social classifications of the United Nations.[2]

In the proposed taxonomy, the IAEA definitions for "competency" and "competence" (IAEA, 2009)[3] have been adopted and competencies have been mapped to one or more of four categories: technical, regulatory, business, and personal (respectively denoted as: T, R, B and P in Tables A4.5-A4.8 of Appendix 4).

Here the focus has been on technical and compliance competencies. It is however stressed that the competencies, training and continuous professional development listed are advisory and do not have regulatory jurisdiction. Further, the examples chosen have been "normalised" for reasons of clarity in terminology and variance that naturally occur across an international sample. It is also stressed that for certain roles (not explicitly stated in this study) there is a requirement for a high-level of security training. Because this taxonomy is not meant to be exhaustive these are excluded.

Importantly, all job profiles are attached to some degree of nuclearisation that determines the education or training requirement as "nuclear-aware", "nuclearised", or "nuclear" (see Figure 1.2).

1. It is noted in this connection that guidelines to selection criteria for key nuclear roles in nuclear power plants and in nuclear research reactors are published by the IAEA (2001).

2. www.ilo.org/public/english/bureau/stat/isco/.

3. "Competencies are knowledge, skills and attitudes in a particular field, which, when acquired, allow a person to perform a job or task to identified standards." "Competence is the ability to put the competencies (i.e. skills, knowledge and attitudes) into practice in order to perform activities or a job in an effective and efficient manner within an occupation or position to identified standards." (IAEA, 2009).

Of highest priority in all aspects of workforce development has been the embedding of a safety culture, as is consistent with all nuclear policy and regulatory developments at both national and international level. The degree of nuclearisation required within a sector, and the corresponding size of the corresponding workforce strata are illustrated through the "competence pyramid" depicted in Chapter 1.

### 3.2.3 An illustrative taxonomy – The workforce in nuclear power plants

In Appendix 4 an illustrated example is also provided to exemplify the derivation of detailed job specifications.

*NPP sectors*

The sectors are defined as:

- **NPP new build** (NPP-NB) – planning, design, construction, commissioning and handover of the licensed plant;
- **NPP operation** (NPP-O) – electricity generation, including outages for inspection and maintenance;
- **NPP decommissioning** (NPP-D) – the removal of nuclear materials and the dismantling of the plant so that the site can be delicensed or reused.

*NPP functions*

Each sector, as defined above, has been sub-categorised into four functions. Functions may apply to more than one activity and even more than one sector. For instance, the activity of radiation protection sits within the safety and environment function of both NPP-O and NPP-D but would also reside in the design function of NPP-NB.

For **NPP new build**, the key functions assigned are, in sequence: *design*, *supply*, *construction* and *commission*. These are delivered by personnel working within a project team, whether as part of the owner-operator company, or with a contractor. These functions appear successively in an NPP-NB so that the composition of the project team changes over the time frame of NPP-NB.

The details of each function are briefly illustrated below.

*The NPP-NB design function* of the nuclear plant requires multidisciplinary teams which must provide the function of a safe and efficient design of the nuclear plant, including:

- the specification of components and aspects of the plant;
- the design of the reactor, its nuclear fuel and the surrounding plant to meet a wide range of normal operating (steady state as well as transients) and fault conditions, and including the defined radiological limits in all areas of the plant along with the complement of personnel required to work in controlled areas;
- the safety/security analyses of the plant that must achieve acceptance by the regulator to gain the operating licence.

*The NPP-NB supply function* incorporates the equipment and structures which are installed to form the plant. These are typically procured from the supply chain of a client or project organisation.

*The NPP-NB construction function* embraces all activities on the site, including civil works, and plant installation prior to start-up and "cold" commission of equipment.

*The NPP-NB commission function* of the nuclear plant takes place in three stages. In stage 1, commissioning of the reactors and associated equipment and systems takes place in the absence of the nuclear fuel. In stage 2, the fuel is loaded and the commissioning focus is to confirm core design, e.g. reactivity values for the in-core mechanisms such as control rods. In stage 3, the integrated plant is commissioned up to and including full power operation.

For **NPP operation** the key functions assigned must be maintained in parallel for the duration of the operating life of the plant. These are *operations, maintenance, waste management, safety and environment*.

The complexity of safety and compliance within NPP-O demands a high degree of nuclearisation of the resident workforce.

*The NPP-O operation function* defines the running of the plant to produce electricity. It starts with handover from commissioning. Once this is completed the plant is licensed to raise power and commercial operation can begin. Operations then remain in control of the plant until this has been shut down at end of its life (which may be up to 60 years). After a "cool down" phase of a few years, and when removal of the cooled fuel is complete, the site formally goes into decommissioning.

*The NPP-O maintenance function* defines all activities necessary to keep the plant in operational order, subject to receiving permission to carry out the necessary work.

*The NPP-O waste management function* defines the collection and packaging of radioactive wastes of all kinds on the nuclear site for its safe storage and, ultimately, its removal under licence from the site at an appropriate and appointed stage, as required.

*The NPP-O safety and environment function* defines all safety assessments and activities necessary to ensure the safe operation of the plant at all times. The safety and environment function advises all other functions on aspects such as work in controlled areas and records of radioactive dosage of all personnel on the site.

For **NPP decommissioning** the key functions include a comprehensive nuclear and non-nuclear organisation. This is essentially NPP-NB in reverse but complicated by the presence of radioactivity. As with NPP-NB, the functions define the work demands of a project organisation (a team working to reduce risk, remove redundant facilities and clear a site for future use). Although the approach is more akin to NPP-NB than NPP-O, the functions themselves are more closely aligned to those of NPP-O, the sector from whence NPP-D transitions. The key functions are *decommissioning, waste management, maintenance, safety and environment*.

Functions and job roles in NPP-D are phase-dependent. Accordingly, resources and planning are shaped to the requirements of each phase.

*The NPP-D decommissioning function* defines control and execution of the site decommissioning activities at all times from start until the remediated site is handed over for new use.

*The NPP-D maintenance function* defines all activities necessary to keep the decommissioning equipment and processes in working order, subject to permission to work.

*The NPP-D waste management function* defines a major commitment to dealing with large amounts of waste generated, assuming storage of high-level waste during NPP-O phase applies.

*The NPP-D safety and environment function* defines dealing with the changing safety and environmental activities in the changing conditions during phasing out of decommissioning and producing the related safety cases.

### *NPP job roles*

Job roles for NPP are recorded in Appendices 4.[4] As described above, the job roles of design engineer, procurement engineer, resident engineer and commissioning engineer are pivotal job roles to each of the functions. These job roles together with those of mechanical design technician, and trades (process, mechanical and electrical) bring to light the typical nuclear awareness requirements for the contractor workforces (see Appendix 4).

Of particular interest is the degree to which job roles at various occupational levels require nuclearisation. Some high-level considerations are provided below.

4. Actual titles may vary from country to country.

For *NPP-NB design*, there is a large input of nuclear knowledge and experience. The overall safe operation of the plant is managed by safety analysts who provide information which the nuclear regulator will need in order to approve operation of the plant. At the earliest stages of a new build (or, indeed, a plant life-extension project), the design engineer executes the design and provides equipment specifications and drawings to the procurement engineer for supply.

In the *NPP-NB supply function* typically a procurement engineer works with the design engineer to capture the relevant technical and commercial requirements and issues a request for quotation. On receipt of the bids, the procurement engineer performs a commercial evaluation and obtains the technical evaluation from the design engineer, places the order and administers the technical aspects of the contract with assistance from the design engineer.

For *NPP-NB construction* the supplied equipment is delivered to the site where the resident engineer interacts with the design engineer and the site construction workforces to ensure the equipment is accounted for and that it is installed to specifications. As the resident engineering team does not have the full knowledge of the system design or component exceptions and acceptances, the resident engineer will rely on the knowledge of the procurement and design engineers to support resolution of supplier issues during the equipment installation. Handover of the installed system to the commissioning engineer then takes place. In this function there is limited need for nuclear knowledge on the construction site, since no nuclear material will appear until this function is completed. Nevertheless, basic nuclear awareness is essential to understanding the requirement for the highest levels of quality and adherence to specification. The requirement for nuclear knowledge in the construction and commission functions is more stringent, for instance, where works are at a licensed nuclear site with existing nuclear plant operations (e.g. for a plant upgrade), and therefore have nuclear hazards around the work. In such cases the individual may be required to undertake awareness training in regulatory compliance issues such as:

- the safety, security and behavioural expectations of those working on nuclear power plants;
- the fundamental principles and implications of radiation hazards;
- the procedures for dealing with radioactive discharges, waste, environmental control and emergencies;
- the reasons for and application of a variety of safety management systems;
- the implications and relevance of company policies, external legislation and regulation on working practices.

In the *NPP-NB commission function*, the commissioning engineer is responsible for verifying that the system functions to its specification and it is common for the design engineer to sign off on the commission acceptance, assuring that the quality and technical requirements of the system are acceptable for handover to operations.

All NPP-O functions require a team of qualified professionals, technicians and crafts, many of whom become specialists in the nuclear industry. The operation function requires some of the most significant nuclear competencies. Nevertheless, it is common for some of this expertise to be supplemented through contractors for maintenance and refuelling in particular. The size and composition of the NPP-O workforce which is based on site tends not to change over the operating life of the plant in the way that it does for NPP-NB and NPP-D. Indeed, the regulatory body may require a defined workforce complement to be sustained throughout.

Job roles of plant manager, operations manager and technician, control room supervisor, reactor operator, process equipment engineer and technician, mechanical maintenance engineer and technician, fitters, waste operator, and health physics manager, all typify activities in each area (see Tables A4.2 and A4.6).

In the case of *NPP-D*, job roles of different occupational level such as site engineer, decommissioning supervisor and operator, maintenance fitter, radioactive waste operations manager, radioactive waste supervisor, radiation protection team leader and health physics surveyor, and safety case lead author typify activities in each area (see Tables A4.3 and A4.7). Some of the job roles may not be exclusive to the NPP industry (e.g. radiation protection) but most require specific nuclear knowledge. Such roles mostly require, in addition, conventional engineering or technical qualifications and competencies.

### 3.2.4 An illustrative taxonomy – The workforce in nuclear research reactors

*Sectors and functions*

Although the main body of this chapter is concerned with the taxonomy of nuclear power plants, the taxonomy for nuclear research reactors (NRRs) was also considered. This was collated in parallel, as most countries that operate nuclear power plants also have NRR facilities. As NRRs contain nuclear fuel, they are covered by the international treaties on nuclear safety and non-proliferation and by the regulatory licence regime. In addition, many of the radiation safety, security and safeguards regimes apply equally.

The utilisation of RRs is extensive and covers training, research and development, radioisotope production and neutron-based research (see below for some detail). As a result the instrumentation and control features lend a uniqueness to individual design, operation and power rating of a given research reactor. In addition, the lack of standardisation of designs and flexibility adds complexity to the competency requirements. For low powered RRs, training and education as well as research form the main utilisation categories. Medium and high powered reactors tend to handle specialised research within their designed utilisation. Driven by costs and increasing technological sophistication, RRs are evolving into three categories: educational RRs, quasi-commercial RRs and advanced application RRs.

Although it would be consistent to align the NRR sectors with those of NPP-NB, O and D, this has not proved practical for this taxonomy, because of the smaller scale of both deployment and employment. Given the diversity and specialisation required by the utilisation, NRR has been retained as a single sector. This has been achieved by: *i)* referring to NPP-NB for supply and construction of an NRR; *ii)* incorporating design under the function identified as design and engineering; *iii)* including safety with operation in a single operation and control function; *iv)* referring to NPP-D for decommissioning; and *v)* capturing maintenance and waste together under the operation and control function. The resulting functions are thereby considered to be a good approximation to an operating research reactor.

Three key functions were identified for NRRs; these were developed in cognisance of the IAEA standards in this area. The functions are:

- **NRR design and engineering** – Similar to NPP-O but on a smaller scale. An interdependency between design and engineering is the intended utilisation. The design must therefore embrace this at the outset.
- **NRR utilisation** – Utilisation gives the reactor its purpose and the activities will, accordingly, depend on the nature of the utilisation. This may require, for instance, special engineering such as: the installation of specialised beam tubes, of irradiation thimbles in-core, or the installation measurement devices for particular purposes.
- **NRR operations and control** – The demands for utilisation must be balanced with the constraints of operation. This must always be within the authorised limits for the reactor. Control in this context includes safety and waste management activities, which are similar to NPP-O but on a smaller scale, with specialist consideration due to the uniqueness that utilisation may present.

*Job roles*

The level of detail in the organisational structure and staffing may change considerably for different types of reactors and their power levels, and be substantially reduced for low power RRs and for reactors with limiting characteristics (e.g. with very low excess reactivity or a large negative temperature coefficient). Representative job roles are listed in Appendix 4. Because of the diversity of NRR facilities three of the most common job roles, reactor manager, reactor operator and radiation protection officer, have been chosen as detailed examples in Appendix 4 (Tables A4.4 and A4.8).

 NUCLEAR EDUCATION AND TRAINING: FROM CONCERN TO CAPABILITY, ISBN 978-92-64-17637-9, © OECD 2012

For **design and engineering**, given the wide variety of power levels, modes of operation and uses, differences in siting and operating organisations, the designs of RR facilities exhibit significant differences in terms of configurations. Typically, workers concerned with the design of RRs represent a very small portion of the NRR workforce. Furthermore, as the intended reactor utilisation is determinant on the design, a strong interface between the two functions is required. The conceptual and detailed design, integration and qualification of devices, calculation tools and simulation models will have to comply with the end user needs as well as the reactor safety and environment.

Within **reactor utilisation**, a key position is the utilisation manager, responsible for the interface between the operating organisation and utilisation customers and ultimately accountable for the integration of irradiation programmes so that safe operation and utilisation of the research reactor are ensured. Among other utilisation roles for which general training requirements should be designated are: utilisation operator and supervisor, laboratory technicians and utilisation scheduler. For experimenters or other users who have been granted access to the RR facility, at least basic training in radiation protection and emergency response should be imparted, commensurate with their responsibilities and conditions of access to the reactor building (IAEA, 2008).

Under **operations and control**, the operating personnel consist of the reactor manager, reactor operator and other individuals involved in the operation, maintenance and, in some cases, use of the reactor. Their responsibilities include, *inter alia*, implementation of the safety policy of the operating organisation, establishment and fostering of a safety culture, and control and verification of safety related activities. The reactor manager has direct responsibility for all aspects of the operation, utilisation and modification of the reactor. In discharging this responsibility, the reactor manager should also be responsible for the overall co-ordination of technical support functions and for the qualification (including adequate initial training and continuing training) of the operating personnel (IAEA, 2008).

### 3.2.5 *An illustrative taxonomy – The workforce in nuclear regulation*

Regulators are a unique part of the workforce by force of their statutory powers in each country with NPP or NRR facilities. The key functions (in taxonomy parlance) of a regulatory body are described in detail in each country's nuclear legislature. It was found that the degree of variation and interpretation in this sector did not lend itself to full classification in this taxonomy. It is worth noting, however, that the IAEA has published extensively on safety standards and, in particular, regulatory matters.[5]

Four key functions of NR that are *normally* present are:

- **NR assessment and review** – Each country maintains a regulatory body with the legal authority to grant licences and to regulate the siting, design, construction, commissioning, operation and decommissioning of nuclear installations.
- **NR authorisation** – Authorisation displays the greatest diversity. It can entail the expected licensing, certification or registration – including responsible personnel working in the health physics departments of nuclear installations – but it can also comprise approval of equipment or manufactures and licensing/certification of personnel (IAEA, 2001b).
- **NR inspection and enforcement** – The regulatory body conducts inspections to independently check the operator and the state of the facility and to provide a high-level of confidence of the operator's compliance (as detailed above). In addition to technical, safety and environmental specifications and management systems, the regulatory body also requires that appropriate processes are in place to ensure that the licensee/operating organisation has assured the competence of its workforce. In this context training usually refers to in-house training at the licensee's training centre.

5. www-ns.iaea.org/standards/.

- **NR regulation and guidance** – Advice and guidance in requirements and expectations to operators and to government and the public on compliance and radiation control, e.g. over emissions, etc.

In addition, supplementary functions such as emergency preparedness and technical support may also rest with the regulatory body.

## 3.3 Analysis

### *3.3.1 Nuclear job role specifications*

This section undertakes an analysis of commonalities in the various job role specifications. The findings reported hereby lay the basis for the recommendations summarised in Chapter 4.

Over 100 key job roles have been identified to illustrate the taxonomy. These are summarised in Appendix 4. Thirty roles in NPP and NRR have been refined in Appendix 4 (Tables A4.5 to A4.8). At least one job specification is present for each function of each NPP sector. Of the 30 detailed job specifications, 14 relate to professional roles, 10 to technical roles, and 6 to craft roles. Of the craft specifications, two are grouped for nuclear relevance. In this way, the role of trades of NPP-NB covers mechanical, electrical and process engineering trades. By the same consideration, the role of nuclear maintenance fitter of NPP-D covers mechanical, electrical and instrumentation trades.

As illustrated in Figure 3.3, the specifications capture job title, description, entry-level qualifications and experience, occupational levels, competencies, continuous professional development and training. It is unsurprising to find some international convergence in the job titles and descriptions, as the industry has become more commercial and global. This is also a manifestation of international co-operation and guidelines of global nuclear organisations. Consistency also holds for the occupational levels of professional, technical and craft and their corresponding entry-level qualifications being, normally, higher education, vocational education with experience, and secondary education combined with vocational development respectively. It is in the entry-level qualifications, and to some extent vocational qualifications, where variance appears, driven by legacy, policy and terminology differences between nations. This has been "normalised" across the taxonomy by retaining only the most commonly accepted terms for the supply of qualifications.

Despite the range of legislative and regulatory frameworks within the contributing sample, there is also much common ground in the competencies. In general, a high-level of competence, qualification and training is required for all the jobs identified. With respect to competencies, it emerges, unsurprisingly, that the competencies, which are defining to the sector, belong to the technical and the regulatory categories, with the personal and business categories being the most generic. Consequently, the technical and regulatory competencies are highly defined and are bounded largely by requirements for capability, safety and compliance.

It is in defining continuous professional development and training related to each job specification where the greatest variation was found in style, description and detail, which were "normalised" for general alignment.

### *3.3.2 Competence assurance*

Despite the "normalisation" that has been undertaken in the job profiles examined, identified continuous professional development and training varies in detail, although there is a discernable core of nuclear safety, technical and regulatory compliance and nuclear security. In the absence of a recognised competence assurance framework, this variation leads to diversity of company training policies and the provision of training in response to demand for such. To some extent this is appropriate and allows scope for local interpretation. On a broader consideration, the absence of a recognised competence assurance framework and the attendant standards for nuclear jobs may lead to diversity and inconsistency in appointments, in training and thereby to restricted mobility of workforces in the global supply chain. The discussion below illustrates how, in the absence of standards for training, this diversity may continue.

 NUCLEAR EDUCATION AND TRAINING: FROM CONCERN TO CAPABILITY, ISBN 978-92-64-17637-9, 

From the utilities to their vendors and manufacturers together with the civil and engineering construction companies and the extended supply chain, variation in training (including continuous professional development) can be due to: company in-house training capability, company outsourcing policy, and the nuclear context of the business of the company. These factors are elaborated below.

### *In-house training*

Capability in this area is commonly related to company size. The larger the company the more likely it is to have HR and training policies and the expertise to deliver an in-house training programme.

### *Outsourced training*

The "provider" of training in this context above may be: an educational institution, a private training company, a contractor providing a technical service, an equipment supplier or vendor (e.g. Areva or Westinghouse), or an organisation such as a professional body, industry body or august agency, association or authority, etc. In this respect, the IAEA maintains an *Electronic Nuclear Training Catalogue*.[6] Representative international examples of such training are:

- for regulation, operation, safety assessment and RRs the *International Atomic Energy Agency Nuclear Safety Standards Training Modules*;[7]
- for engineering, the American Society of Mechanical Engineers offers a comprehensive Training and Development Programme;[8]
- for nuclear power professionals, INPO[9] has created a set of training requirements for control room operators and several other classifications of workers.

Key determinants in employer choice of training are suitability, regulation, accessibility and affordability of the training on offer by external providers.

Accessibility will be determined by consideration of choice in terms of the location of provider, the delivery and support strategies of the training provision, and the flexibility of the provision to cope with the availability of personnel.

Affordability will be determined by consideration of value in relation to the cost of the provision. In some cases the cost of training may be included in the technical service of the contractor and assessment of the training may have formed part of the business relationship. Where training is an additional cost of employment, the value of the training will be a complex business decision for the employer. On the other hand, the cost of training will arise from a complex pricing assessment by the training provider. Typically this will include consideration of the prestige of the provider, the technical level the training is designed to, the size of the cohort being trained, the time frame for delivery, the delivery strategy, competitor analysis, "kitemarks" of excellence, and the prices that the market will bear.

### *Nuclear context*

Training may be driven by regulation; it may also be a contractual requirement from an operator to its supply chain as part of competence assurance or regulatory compliance. The nature and extent of the training will also be attributed, to a large degree, by the proximity of the personnel to the nuclear island.

6. http://entrac.iaea.org/Login.aspx.
7. www.nucleus.iaea.org/CIR/CIR/NSS.html.
8. http://files.asme.org/asmeorg/Education/Europe/Courses/23861.pdf.
9. www.inpo.info/AboutUs.htm.

It is clear, therefore, that the "market" in training is a complex and a sophisticated one. While much detailed information advice and guidance on training for nuclear operators has been published by the IAEA (e.g. IAEA, 2002) there is scope for more widespread accreditation of training to cogently direct employer choices, especially where training is outsourced.

It is in the large and transient contractor workforces where clarity, conformity and reliability in sourcing appropriate training may be of particular value in order to be safe, credible and compliant. (In this instance "transient" could mean 5-7 years on a new build site, weeks on an operating site during a maintenance outage, or years on a decommissioning site.)

The nuclear operating companies which are responsible for their qualified workers ultimately drive the market in training. Nuclear operators take a measured risk approach to competence assurance throughout the supply chain. This is no more than normal business practice in any field, e.g. as in quality assurance or customer service. The stakes are higher, though, for nuclear. The technical demands and the regulated safety culture heighten the consequences of non-conformance. Through responsibility to their customers (the paying public and general commerce) and the regulator, nuclear operators can require the highest standards of training in their supply chain and could direct suppliers to accredited training as part of competence assurance.

The ad hoc expert group supporting this work strongly believes that management systems that capture and assure competence are highly desirable. Competence assurance guidelines are thereby key. Lessons learnt from various nuclear projects testify to the complexity of competence assurance from the operator through to the supply chain.

Effective accreditation of training can provide the confidence required for credibility and compliance and should lead to enhanced safety. It could lead to mutual recognition of workers among potential employers, including those operating in a global context. Academic accreditation is a common practice in education and is a culture that could be carried over to training. In the United States accredited training programmes are a regulatory requirement, but this only covers the accredited utility and their workers. Although some competencies and knowledge are generic and can be transferred, there remains plant specific training that is prerequisite for each worker at a particular site.

Accreditation of training does not exist in most other countries. To achieve this, the development of occupational standards against job roles would be required, or more effectively, cognate families of job roles as categorised by a taxonomy. While nuclear operators set requirements related to the education, training and experience of personnel operating and maintaining nuclear facilities and equipment consistently with safety standards and guidance set by the IAEA (e.g. IAEA, 2002 and 2008) or national standards, such requirements present a good deal of variability in different countries.

In this connection, the Bologna Process provides for the alignment of higher education qualification structures across the European Union.[10] ABET does the same within the United States and elsewhere. While Bologna is aimed at providers of education *and not* employers, the process has at heart the principles of setting a common baseline of academic knowledge and of mobility. This in itself, however, does not provide for the specific occupational standards for the nuclear workforce.

Returning to the nuclear industry, some countries have adopted independently administered Nuclear Passport (United Kingdom),[11] *Carnet d'accès* (France), *Qual Cards* (United States) schemes for the contractor community. In the EC, the ECVET is aimed at facilitating the transfer, recognition and accumulation of assessed learning outcomes of individuals on their way to achieving a qualification and ultimately to the ambition of a competence-based European Passport or portfolio of learning outcomes.[12] In relation to this, the EHRO-N has recently launched an ECVET-oriented job

10. http://ec.europa.eu/education/higher-education/doc1290_en.htm.
11. www.nuclearskillspassport.co.uk/.
12. www.cedefop.europa.eu/EN/news/8987.aspx.

taxonomy in the nuclear area.[13] In the United States, INPO has established training guidelines and requirements for the key jobs at all operating plants, including reactor operators, plant engineers, and technicians. Every nuclear operator must have an accredited training programme that follows a well defined strategic approach to training and strict adherence to the knowledge and skills requirements outlined in relevant INPO "ACAD" documents. Accreditation is performed by the independent National Nuclear Accrediting Board. A new development in the United States to assist in the recruitment of new entry level personnel is the Nuclear Uniform Curriculum Programme[14] (NUCP) which is an example of partnership between the industry and technical (two year) colleges. The NUCP supplies, through academic courses, fundamental knowledge which would otherwise be delivered in utility training programmes, thereby expediting the time needed in training by the new employee before becoming job task qualified.

The benefit of such accreditation systems is in their common trajectory towards recognition and standardisation of qualifications and training between various companies. This, in turn, facilitates commonality in regulatory compliance, competence assurance, workforce mobility and the avoidance of repetitive preparatory training at different company sites or by successive employers adding efficacy in competence assurance.

On the international stage a number of prominent training developments have taken place in recent years. These noteworthy developments have emerged separately and are largely underpinned by the recognised need of independent recognition and accreditation. The main protagonists in this area are nuclear organisations, employers and university networks, such as the previously noted INPO in the United States and, internationally, the IAEA, WANO and, among others:

- the World Nuclear University[15] – a joint venture between WNA, IAEA, OECD/NEA, and WANO;
- the European Nuclear Leadership Academy;[16]
- the European Nuclear Education Network.[17]

One area that has moved closer to mutual recognition and accreditation on an international basis is radiological protection. The European Network on Education and Training in Radiological Protection (ENETRAP) is a network of universities developing internationally accredited training for radiological protection professionals.[18]

Concurrently to this work, a number of examples of nuclear taxonomy in action have emerged (two of these are illustrated in some detail in Appendix 5).

Our analysis of the operation and impact of each taxonomy underlines the importance of an independent body for the accreditation of training. INPO provides this for training programmes in the United States and South Africa. The National Skills Academy, Nuclear is growing in this capacity in the United Kingdom. For the future, adoption of nuclear training accreditation may be considered more widely. Initiatives in this direction are already taking place at the European level.

Another observation emerging from the analysis of the taxonomy is the international consensus on the need for "raw" components of basic nuclear training covering fundamental technical and regulatory matters. This would support the production of an outline programme in "basic nuclear industry awareness" that would have application across all sectors.

13. http://publications.jrc.ec.europa.eu/repository/handle/111111111/22304.
14. www.nei.org/careersandeducation/nuclear-uniform-curriculum-program.
15. www.world-nuclear-university.org/.
16. www.enela.eu/.
17. www.enen-assoc.org/.
18. www.sckcen.be/enetrap/.

## References

EC (2009), *Nuclear Safety in a Situation of Fading Nuclear Experience*, European Commission, Brussels, Belgium.

IAEA (1991), *Safety Culture, a Report by the International Nuclear Safety Advisory Group*, INSAG-4, IAEA, Vienna, Austria. Available at www-pub.iaea.org/MTCD/publications/PDF/Pub882_web.pdf.

IAEA (2001), *Assuring the Competence of Nuclear Power Plant Contractor Personnel*, IAEA, Vienna, Austria. Available at www-pub.iaea.org/MTCD/publications/PDF/te_1232_prn.pdf.

IAEA (2001a), *Applications of Probabilistic Safety Assessment (PSA) for Nuclear Power Plants*, IAEA, Vienna, Austria. Available at www-pub.iaea.org/MTCD/publications/PDF/te_1200_prn.pdf

IAEA (2001b), *Training the Staff of the Regulatory Body for Nuclear Facilities: A Competency Framework*, IAEA, Vienna, Austria. Available at www-ns.iaea.org/downloads/ni/training/rgbd_trg.pdf.

IAEA (2002), *Recruitment, Qualification and Training of Personnel for Nuclear Power Plants*, IAEA Safety Guide No. NS-G-2.8, IAEA, Vienna, Austria. Available at www-pub.iaea.org/MTCD/publications/PDF/Pub1140_scr.pdf.

IAEA (2006), *Code of Conduct for the Operation and Utilization of Research Reactors*, IAEA, Vienna, Austria. Available at www-pub.iaea.org/MTCD/publications/PDF/CODEOC-RR_web.pdf.

IAEA (2008), *The Operating Organisation and the Recruitment, Training and Qualification of Personnel for Research Reactors*, IAEA Safety Guide No. NS-G-4.5, IAEA, Vienna, Austria. Available at www-pub.iaea.org/MTCD/publications/PDF/Pub1335_web.pdf.

IAEA (2009), *Managing Human Resources in the Field of Nuclear Energy*, IAEA, Vienna, Austria. Available at www-pub.iaea.org/MTCD/Publications/PDF/Pub1397_web.pdf

IAEA (2011), *Status and Trends in Nuclear Education*, IAEA, Vienna, Austria. Available at www-pub.iaea.org/MTCD/publications/PDF/P1475_web.pdf.

IAEA (2012), *Power Reactor Information System*, IAEA, Vienna, Austria. Available at www.iaea.org/programmes/a2/.

NEA (2000), *Nuclear Education and Training: Cause for Concern?*, OECD, Paris, France.

NEA (2008), *Nuclear Energy Outlook*, Nuclear Energy Agency, OECD, Paris, France.

SNE-TP (2010), *Current and Future Uses of Nuclear Infrastructure in Europe, SNE-TP* – Working Group ETKM – Subgroup 4, available at www.enen-assoc.org/data/document/2010-report_etkm_gr4_final.pdf.

*Chapter 4*

# Ensuring capability – the recommendations

## 4.1 Nuclear human resource features and requirements

Achieving a steady and sustainable workforce supply for the nuclear sector is a challenge not only because of the high numbers involved globally, but also because of the high-level of competency required of its workers. The distinctive features characterising nuclear energy and its applications necessitate very high overall skills in both operations and management, and accordingly, strict requirements for E&T.

The nuclear workforce has been classified in three categories of personnel for the purposes of training and development: the "nuclear" (the specialist), the "nuclearised" (the experienced) and the "nuclear-aware" (the locally inducted employment). The "nuclear" and the "nuclearised" are most prominent in employment on nuclear licensed sites; the third is most prominent in the significant contractor supply chain (see Figure 1.2).

At the top of the pyramid, for the smaller group of high-level professionals, the competence acquisition route is fundamentally through academic qualifications, with in-depth knowledge achieved through long periods of specialised education and/or experience. This was the focus of the previous NEA study. Moving towards the base of the pyramid, competency development shifts to training, focused on a particular job, task or set of tasks. Many previous reports have focused on the top levels, where academic training has been of high importance, seeking to assess the supply and demand for these types of workers. This provides a strong link between this type of training and the capacities of universities and other training institutes. However, few reports consider how to provide a comprehensive approach to training across the range required to cover the full pyramid or how this range of training should occur. In this report, the ad hoc expert group has looked at a way forward in identifying training requirements and in assessing the availability of facilities that could provide practical training.

Recent industry workforce surveys have shown that in some countries, the larger part of the nuclear workforce at the base of the pyramid constitutes the greatest near-term workforce need, confronting the nuclear community with a new challenge. While since *Cause for Concern* little co-ordinated effort has been directed at technical and crafts, increasing attention will be required for the training and "nuclearisation" of these levels.

Owing to the long period of stasis in new civilian programmes the nuclear community still faces multiple challenges, with a large impending retirement of the ageing workforce, the significant and persistent attrition experienced in the field, and a decline in the pool of people with recent construction experience. Strains in nuclear HR supply remain high and concerns over the adequacy of nuclear E&T still prevail in the international arena.

Bearing in mind the long lead times generally required for nuclear E&T, the establishment and preservation of an adequate nuclear workforce supply calls for systematic planning decades ahead.

In this respect, contradictory energy policies can have grave effects. A deteriorated global context caused by the persistent financial crisis and the negative sentiments in the wake of the Fukushima Daiichi accident heighten uncertainties and may exacerbate existing shortcomings. Indeed, shifting or deferred government decisions act as deterrent mechanisms in investment and employment, and have deleterious repercussions on the interest and engagement of younger people in the industry.

This is grafted on a situation in science and engineering which is, by and large, already weak. Although student recruitment in nuclear has, in a few countries, turned positive as a result of favourable occupational prospects and a greater understanding of energy and environmental needs, typically, in most countries, the young generation still tends to avoid or leave technical and scientific disciplines across all areas.

Thus, a coherent intervention by governments, industry, universities and research and development organisations remains vital to avert the risk of manpower shortages in some countries and maintain the stock of a skilled and competent workforce. This is necessary in order to keep a flow of new recruits which is sustainable in the long term and, in particular, adequate to offset impending retirement.

## 4.2 Ten years on – the developments

Looking at developments over the past decade, evidence from countries suggests that, in response to the persisting concerns and new market conditions, stakeholders have taken actions, albeit not immediate and often driven by "environmental" or external determinants. Challenges have been acknowledged and progress has been achieved in addressing certain issues and recommendations raised in *Cause for Concern* (NEA, 2000). However, overall, concerns remain over the fact that a process for providing a sustainable HR supply has not been achieved in all countries.

Alongside the outstanding challenges, the box below lists initiatives and examples of good practice reported by different stakeholders, while some of the most prominent are discussed in more detail in the relevant chapters of the report.

| Stakeholder | What is working well | Challenges |
|---|---|---|
| Governments | Government support, policies and strategic planning (in some countries).<br>Governments funding support to HRD (in some countries).<br>The development of national networks.<br>The sustained international co-operation and exchange.<br>The establishment of ad hoc bodies (such as CFEN in France, the UK Cogent Sector Skills Council and its Nuclear Employers Steering Group and the Nuclear Human Resources Development Council in Japan).<br>Systematic approach to address the workforce shortage (including periodic and comprehensive assessments of needs).<br>Government support for student and university research. | Too few governments engaged.<br>Lack of long-term vision for existing programmes.<br>Fluctuating policies in several member countries.<br>Inconsistent/inadequate support in others.<br>The dilemma and difficulties in sustaining national education and training infrastructure, in countries where smaller numbers of specialists are required. |
| Universities | Industry, educational and research institutions working together – even better when the government is involved.<br>Development of some highly integrated programmes.<br>Progress towards standardisation and accreditation to favour recognition and mobility.<br>Train the trainers programmes.<br>Innovative learning.<br>Development of platforms listing available educational programmes.<br>International networks and international collaboration. | What are the standards? Industry/academia, different length, breath, residency and input qualifications.<br>How to harmonise and keep the standards?<br>Introduction of elements of safety culture.<br>"Nuclearisation" training of non-nuclear professionals.<br>Introduction and early training on elements of non-technical knowledge and skills (e.g. managerial skills, "social-related" subjects, law, economics, finance, business, etc.).<br>Language barriers.<br>More hands on training needed.<br>Instructors at all levels need practical experience. |

 NUCLEAR EDUCATION AND TRAINING: FROM CONCERN TO CAPABILITY, ISBN 978-92-64-17637-9, © OECD 2012

| Stakeholder | What is working well | Challenges |
|---|---|---|
| Industry | Making concerted efforts with other sectors.<br>Opening training courses to others and in an international context.<br>In various instances making resources available for education:<br>– working with academic institutions e.g. internships, scholarships, funding of chairs;<br>– getting involved in shaping and delivering courses;<br>– partnering with local universities and community colleges.<br>Using varied pedagogical tools (simulators, mock-ups, etc.).<br>Pursuing active recruitment and outreach to students, teachers and media.<br>Working towards standardisation and the recognition of unified curriculum programmes. | Safety culture is difficult to measure, establish and maintain.<br>Few multinational suppliers – confronted with many different standards and codes.<br>Reluctance of some industry to make research facilities available for students.<br>Networks such as those developed for educational programmes should be expanded to cover also technical training (some existing networks such as UNENE and ENEN are considering expanding their scope to train technical personnel).<br>External and internal attrition. |
| Research institutes | Research institutes are promoting high profile research projects.<br>Co-ordinating with universities and other stakeholders:<br>– offering internships, scholarships, awards;<br>– making experts available to guide students and for professorships;<br>– providing transnational access of infrastructures for E&T.<br>Implementing web-based education and training programmes.<br>Promoting joint research initiatives with the industry and universities (pooling resources when these are limited). | Ageing of facilities.<br>Difficulties in replacing them due to:<br>– more stringent regulatory requirements and related operational issues;<br>– uncertainties in financing.<br>High age distribution of experts in research institutes.<br>Lack of innovative training methods.<br>Unclear or changing government policies on research. |

### 4.2.1 *Governments*

In many countries the educational system is shaped by governments. Hence, while actions by other stakeholders are important, without strong government participation, there is limited ability to change the educational system. However, across the board, governments have, in general, done very little of a longer-term and more strategic nature.

Experience shows that active monitoring of demand and supply capacity is a fundamental step for HRD; but, in order for it to bear effective and long-lasting benefits, it should be conducted on an ongoing basis, with assessments undertaken regularly and frequently for systematic planning.

In several countries governments have commissioned manpower assessments. In some cases, the results and recommendations drawn from such surveys triggered significant government actions to address emerging gaps. National councils and bodies have been established (e.g. in France, Japan and in the United Kingdom) to undertake labour market research and workforce planning, which has often proven effective for the initiation of government actions towards human resource development.

Some governments have provided specific support to university programmes and research, which has contributed, in a few instances, to reversing the declining trends of subscription in nuclear engineering. In the United States, evidence shows that the government funding of nuclear education can be tied directly to graduation of students focused on nuclear majors. In years when government funding for scholarships, fellowships, university research and trade schools has been lean, student interest has declined.

In many cases, fluctuating policies or lack of long-term vision for existing programmes leave countries with HRD planning approach and systems which are deficient, inconsistent or inadequate, if not completely absent.

**Recommendation 1**

*Governments should show a continuous and stable engagement in human resource development planning for the long-term timescales that transcend fluctuations in economic cycles. Government involvement should include regular, active monitoring of demand and supply capacity, as well as allocation of funds to support educational programmes which provide a means of developing and maintaining specialist expertise.*

### 4.2.2 Education

Universities have striven for improvements over the last ten years, with some new and advanced nuclear courses being launched in an increasingly global context. In some cases, and notably when assisted by governmental funding and support, academic programmes have succeeded in reversing the declining trend of student recruitments experienced during the 1980s and 1990s.

Healthier numbers of students have also been attracted by the prospect of new build, or high profile research topics and international projects.

Co-ordinating efforts has again proved to be an effective means for the promotion or preservation of nuclear programmes. Academic institutions have realised this, sometime in conjunction with other parties (e.g. research centres), through the establishment of networks, the launch of international programmes, or through the amalgamation of courses, which has been vital in countries with fading nuclear programmes or with a small demand for specialists.

Noteworthy is the creation in some countries of inter-university consortia and college partnerships, allowing early interaction with young students. Universities have engaged with technical colleges to address the increasing demand of craft and technical levels. Sometimes courses are franchised, modular/work-based foundation degrees have been created, vocational training sessions rolled out, some specifically devised for the "nuclearisation" of non-nuclear professionals.

However, in many countries, the supply has not yet reached a sustainable capacity with regard to meeting the demand.

**Recommendation 2**

*Universities should intensify efforts, in collaboration with industry, to provide a greater range of courses and with greater flexibility in means of attendance by students.*

**Recommendation 3**

*Governments should support educational institutions and nuclear technology students at technical colleges to ensure there is a well-rounded workforce available for all of the nuclear careers.*

### 4.2.3 Research

The integration of national research and academic institutes within international frameworks has generally grown. It is widely recognised that a strong and increased participation in international research programmes and the greater involvement of industry in research and training must continue and can considerably improve the attraction of high-calibre students and young researchers in the field.

Co-ordination with universities and other stakeholders has been pursued by research organisations, namely through direct participation on academic curricula, the promotion and delivery of courses and seminars to a varied audience, the offer of internships, the provision of well-equipped laboratories and guidance to domestic and foreign students for their research, the award of prizes, grants and fellowships, the organisation of visits, etc. The involvement of students in MSc theses is also commendable within the limits imposed by the time constraints for both the theses and the research projects.

In assessing the current use and capabilities of nuclear research facilities for E&T purposes, the ad hoc expert group recognises the benefits of a more intensive use of such infrastructure for laboratory sessions. It is through specific hands-on training that safety culture can be crucially instilled in students, who through use of nuclear experimental facilities can be confronted with a real nuclear environment with radiological and physical constraints and where attention to safety becomes a pre-requisite.

Full advantage should be taken of existing facilities, including amenable industry research infrastructure.

### Recommendation 4

*Access to research facilities suitable for education and training purposes should be widened and international co-ordination for such uses should be enhanced. Efforts should be made by governments to financially support existing infrastructure.*

### Recommendation 5

*Research and academic institutions offering laboratory sessions, including computer simulations, should take new initiatives for the collection and preparation of pedagogical materials (books, software) in support of such sessions.*

Computer models and computer simulations do not replace laboratory sessions but can enhance theoretical understanding. The role of simulators in training is mandatory in some countries and is becoming increasingly widespread. Nonetheless, the general view remains that their use in training and education is still to be considered complementary to hands-on training.

### Recommendation 6

*Research facilities should work with industry and academia to create opportunities for more effective use of research facilities so as to enhance education and training.*

NEA, 2004 testified to the deterioration of the financial situation of research institutes, in many countries due to cuts in public funding and to tough competition in the niche market where they sell their services and products. Although this outlook seems to have changed in some countries, with funds being directed to R&D and the support of research infrastructures, concerns have been raised (NEA, 2009 and 2009a) over the fact that many expensive and unique facilities were put into operation in the 1960s. Some of them have already shut down and a substantial number is awaiting the same fate in the next few years.

### Recommendation 7

*Special attention should be directed to the needs of universities for access to relevant nuclear instrumentation and critical facilities, including research reactors to perform research and enhance education. Infrastructure support should be provided to maintain existing nuclear facilities, where these can be refurbished, or to replace them when they are obsolete.*

In this regard, the example of the United States is noted, where the Department of Energy supports over 20 university research reactors and has funded nuclear energy research and equipment upgrades at US colleges and universities.

### 4.2.4 Industry

The engagement of industry has generally been consistent and vigorous across the board. Sometimes this has also led to commendable examples of collaboration with universities and other parties, such as the funding of chairs and sponsoring of educational and research programmes, the direct involvement in the development and delivery of courses, the offer of internships and, in some cases, the opening of research infrastructure to students.

In some countries the industry has also been engaged in the monitoring process of HR demand and supply and has fruitfully partnered with local universities and community colleges to address emerging gaps across different levels.

Of particular notice is the industry participation and initiative in the establishment of multilateral educational networks. The partnership between US utilities and technical colleges has created the Nuclear Uniform Curriculum Program to address the supply of technicians in the United States. Some existing networks such as UNENE and ENEN are considering expanding their scope to train technical personnel, which is deemed to be a worthy development.

#### Recommendation 8

*Networks such as those developed for educational programmes should be expanded to cover technical training as well.*

In the past few years, in the wake of a prospective nuclear renaissance, major industrial players succeeded in ramping-up their recruitment rates worldwide. Most principal industrial actors have developed and maintained strong internal vocational training processes to prepare their personnel and undertake re-staffing. Notably, in some cases, large training centres and programmes have been set up to satisfy the high and diverse recruitment needs. However, as discussed above, attrition is still acute and in some countries the industry has been unable to retain professionals and has suffered the drain of nuclear skills towards other sectors or, in an increasingly globalised context, towards other countries.

Typically, if favourable conditions are instated, careers in the nuclear sector offer the appealing prospect of highly secure and long-term employment, which represents a point of strength of the industry.

#### Recommendation 9

*In order to attract and retain high-calibre young professionals and avert cross-sector and cross-boundary attrition, the industry should provide competitive remuneration, career opportunities and recognition.*

One continual challenge facing the nuclear industry is maintaining and continuously enhancing safety culture. This is difficult to measure, especially when the few multinational suppliers are confronted with many different standards and codes, as well as a global supply chain. Section 4.2.5 develops some further discussions and recommendations on this issue.

### 4.2.5 Internationalisation

A general tendency characterising the sector has been the significant and increasing internationalisation. With a consolidated market of few global technology vendors and progressively more R&D projects developed across national borders, recent years have witnessed an increased globalisation of the civil nuclear industry and its supply chain. Nuclear power has become an international business bounded by international agreements. Greater emphasis has been placed on international collaboration for regulation, precompetitive R&D, as well as the intricate global supply chains involving utilities, vendors and contractors in manufacturing, engineering, construction, operations, maintenance and decommissioning.

Linked to the increased internationalisation, new questions and different issues have emerged, such as student and HR mobility, quality control of education and training, greater understanding


NUCLEAR EDUCATION AND TRAINING: FROM CONCERN TO CAPABILITY, ISBN 978-92-64-17637-9, © OECD 2012

of different typology of nuclear job profiles, and the need for a set of transferable nuclear competencies and safety awareness that support an international supply chain.

On the one hand, this has prompted many international initiatives. The various new programmes of international and intergovernmental bodies have given rise to means by which organisations may source or collaborate on research, education, training and knowledge management at a range of levels internationally, and instruments by which they can also draw from and contribute to labour market research on the supply and demand of human resources in nuclear energy.

Global partnerships committed to enhancing international education and leadership in the peaceful application of nuclear science and technology have been established in the last few years, such as the WNU and the ENELA. The role of the European Commission in supporting HR development has been particularly noteworthy and has resulted in many new collaborative initiatives supporting research and training in nuclear topics (among others: ENEN, the European Fission Training Schemes, EHRO-N and EN3S).

**Recommendation 10**

*Governments should strongly encourage and support international initiatives and programmes, which foster consistent quality of the education and training being delivered in different countries and overall contribute to enhancing human resource development capacities.*

In this new context, in addition to the duties of countries with respect to existing national programmes, there is the emerging responsibility of providers and vendors to develop a competent workforce in recipient countries. Various bilateral and multilateral agreements have been established at different levels (institutional, academic and industrial) and numerous transnational education and training projects have been initiated in several countries. Yet, even with the international components emerging in the nuclear industry and increasingly in education, the responsibility for national education ultimately remains with individual governments.

Countries with strong national nuclear activities, facilities and resources have initiated programmes to "train the trainers", which complement similar programmes conceived by international organisations (notably the International Atomic Energy Agency). These are implemented in close co-operation with interested countries and specifically tailored to their needs and local education systems with the aim of forming a strong pool of indigenous human resources.

The uptake of transnational programmes as well as regional and national networks has often benefitted from improved technological means. Novel communication systems and IT instruments can be more appealing to new generations, and their dissemination has allowed the development of effective and innovative learning methods. Increasingly, web-based resources as well as distance learning are embraced as common practices both by education and research institutions as well as industry training programmes. This has helped to enlarge the pool of prospective students. Through distance learning, students can take courses even when these are not available at their own university, during a semester when they may not be taught, or, importantly, when physical or geographical obstacles would prevent their physical attendance or make it significantly more onerous. However, this raises the issue of consistency and certification.

## 4.3 Approach to developing a common job taxonomy

Recognising this emerging internationalisation of the workforce and the overarching priority to ensure safety, and drawing from the experience of a number of countries, the ad hoc expert group has researched and classified specific examples of job roles with significant nuclear competence that are found across the nuclear industry. This effort lays the basis for the development of a classification system for nuclear job profiles: a framework job taxonomy.

The proposed taxonomic system is of course nominal; it is neither a final nor a unique solution, but it provides a first step to assist the development of classifications.

Nuclear job specifications have been presented for the most typical stages of the lifecycle of a nuclear reactor in power and research, drawing up from the analyses conducted by a number of companies. These may serve as an initial platform on which organisations (nationally or internationally) or individual countries can overlay their own different and specific requirements.

An analysis of commonalities has led to the following findings and recommendations:

- Competence in technical and regulatory matters features consistently and prominently in nuclear job specifications across the globe. Nuclear safety culture is inextricably linked to both.
- Information, advice and guidance on training, especially training on technical and regulatory competencies, could be improved through accreditation of training provision whether it be in-house to a company or outsourced to a provider.
- There are limited international occupational standards to guide nuclear training and workforce development,[1] although there are national standards such as those promulgated by INPO in the United States.[2]
- Apart from the National Nuclear Accreditation Board in the United States and the National Skills Academy in the United Kingdom, there are no other independent national bodies for the accreditation of nuclear training.
- Taxonomy as a tool in workforce development that can aid workforce planning in elaborating scenarios for the supply and demand of skills; in developing training standards, and as a structure for competence assurance management systems such as nuclear passport schemes.
- Both governments and employers can benefit from access to high quality labour market intelligence and training standards. This can inform, for example, targeted policy interventions such as directives on training, or prioritisation on resourcing of higher education and research.
- Dissemination of international guidelines for training and competence assurance would assist employers in choosing or designing appropriate workforce development programmes.

### Recommendation 11

Drawing from the experience of the National Nuclear Accreditation Board in the United States, it is recommended that:

*Consideration should be given to carrying over to training the accreditation and certification culture that is well established in education, and to establishing independent accreditation and certification of training provision and employer schemes.*

Safety culture permeates nuclear job specifications. In this regard, the proposed taxonomy brings into prominence not only the competence assurance considerations of the previous section, but also the technical and regulatory competencies, both of which relate to safety.

### Recommendation 12

There appears to be international consensus on the fundamental components of basic nuclear training covering fundamental technical and regulatory matters to support the production of an outline programme in "basic nuclear awareness" that could have value for the international community. It is therefore recommended that:

*Consideration should be given to the provision of an outline for training in "basic nuclear awareness" with content adequate to cover both the range of nuclear sectors and the range of occupational levels.*

1. It is noted that at a European level there is a strong drive to structuring training and career development across the EU and to establishing European high-quality "reference standards" with the ultimate objective of creating a European competence passport.

2. It is worth noting that the work done by the Institute of Nuclear Power Operations (INPO) for operators is distributed internationally by the World Association of Nuclear Operators (WANO).

 NUCLEAR EDUCATION AND TRAINING: FROM CONCERN TO CAPABILITY, ISBN 978-92-64-17637-9, © OECD 2012

## References

NEA (2000), *Nuclear Education and Training: Cause for Concern?*, OECD, Paris, France.

NEA (2004), *Nuclear Competence Building*, OECD, Paris, France.

NEA (2009), *Research and Test Facilities Required in Nuclear Science and Technology*, OECD, Paris, France.

NEA (2009a), *Support and Test Facilities for Existing and Advanced Reactors* (SFEAR), Report of the Senior Group of Experts on Nuclear Safety Research (SESAR), OECD, Paris, France.

# *Appendix 1* Recommendations from *Nuclear Education and Training: Cause for Concern?*[1]

## 1. The deterioration of nuclear education

### Recommendation

A. We must act now. The actions, described in subsequent recommendations, should be taken up urgently by government, industry, universities, research institutes and the NEA.

## 2. The important role of governments in nuclear education

### Recommendations

A. Governments should engage in strategic energy planning, including consideration of education, manpower and infrastructure.

B. Governments should contribute to, if not take responsibility for, integrated planning to ensure that human resources are available to meet necessary obligations and address outstanding issues.

C. Governments should support, on a competitive basis, young students. They should also provide adequate resources for vibrant nuclear research and development programmes including modernisation of facilities.

D. Governments should provide support by developing "educational networks or bridges" between universities, industry and research institutes.

## 3. The challenges of revitalising nuclear education

### Recommendations

A. Universities should provide basic and attractive educational programmes.

B. Universities should interact early and often with potential students, both male and female, and provide adequate information.

1. NEA, 2000.

## 4. High-quality training needed for staff in industry and research institutes

### Recommendations

A. Industry should continue to provide rigorous training programmes to meet its specific needs.

B. Research institutes need to develop exciting research projects to meet industry's needs and attract quality students and employees.

C. Industry, research institutes and universities need to work together to co-ordinate efforts better to encourage the younger generation.

## 5. Benefits of collaboration and sharing best practices

### Recommendations

A. Member countries should ask the NEA to develop and promote a programme of collaboration between member countries in nuclear education and training.

B. Member countries should ask the NEA to provide a mechanism for sharing best practices in promoting nuclear courses.

## Reference

NEA (2000), *Nuclear Education and Training: Cause for Concern?*, OECD, Paris, France.

# *Appendix 2*
# Country education and training activities

In the 2000 NEA report *Nuclear Education and Training: Cause for Concern?* (NEA, 2000) a few recommendations to governments, universities, research institutes and industry are listed. After ten years, the NEA ETKM expert group has undertaken a review on how and to what extent these recommendations have been addressed. An overview of the initiatives taken by countries is provided below for those NEA member states represented in the group.

# Australia

## Introduction

Nuclear power is not part of the present energy mix in Australia, neither does the current government foresee its introduction in the future.

Nonetheless, as a major supplier of uranium, Australia has historically developed vast experience in the utilisation of research reactors (HIFAR and MOATA, currently shut down) and, more recently, in planning, licensing, construction, commissioning and operation of OPAL research reactor. There are a number of active nuclear research programmes at the Australian Nuclear Science and Technology Organisation (ANSTO) in various institutions, notably the national centre for nuclear science and technology, responsible for delivering specialised advice, scientific services and products to government, industry, academia and other research organisations.

## Government activities

There is no co-ordinated national approach to nuclear education and training (E&T). Government plays no direct role in nuclear education, with minimal investment being allocated in nuclear education over the last 20 years.

A major review: the *Uranium Mining, Processing and Nuclear Energy Review* (UMPNER) (Commonwealth of Australia, 2006) commissioned by the government, was published in 2007. The review found that significant additional human resources would be needed to expand nuclear fuel cycle beyond uranium mining and recommended that nuclear human resource development should be part of government planning and that substantially greater investment and spending should be dedicated to it.

## University activities

A 2006 survey (IEAust, 2006) found a lack of tertiary education in nuclear science and technology in engineering departments in Australian universities. No comprehensive nuclear engineering courses are provided in Australia. Only a few courses are delivered in nuclear physics as part of broader syllabus and, in particular, for medical and health physics applications. Notably, the Australian National University (ANU) conducts research in nuclear physics and fusion systems and imparts postgraduate education in nuclear science. ANU has recently introduced a Master in Nuclear Science and looks to partner with other selected universities to broaden the scope and extend its reach.

Co-ordination is provided by the Australian Institute of Nuclear Science and Engineering (AINSE), a body established in 1958, which has a mandate to train scientific research workers and award scientific research studentships in nuclear science and engineering fields. In June 2006, AINSE has decided to facilitate the formation of an Australia-wide nuclear science and technology school to provide education in a wide range of nuclear related matters from technical aspects of the fuel cycle and reactor operation through nuclear safety and public awareness to political matters of interest to policy makers (Commonwealth of Australia, 2006).

The *Uranium Mining, Processing and Nuclear Energy Review* (Commonwealth of Australia, 2006) highlighted the potential benefits of developing a national educational network involving Australian universities and colleges, industry and ANSTO and, furthermore, the building of alliances with education providers or networks overseas to provide a mechanism for overcoming difficulties with expanding local education and training efforts.

## Industry/research institute activities

The industry has played a primary role in delivering training programmes, promoting resourcing, networking, research (e.g. ANSTO-OPAL) and education (funding chairs). ANSTO provides internal training to meet its own needs for nuclear professionals. At present, the necessary skills are developed through a combination of specialist courses and on-the-job training (IEAust, 2006). However, a situation of crisis persists. Due to the dearth of nuclear experts qualified nationally, in certain technical divisions, every person recruited has come from overseas. In addition, ageing of senior experts is clearly becoming an issue and it is not apparent to what extent younger experts from Australia may be able to fill the gaps at their retirement.

ANSTO operates the world-class multipurpose OPAL research reactor which produces medical isotopes and supplies irradiation services. Research conducted in OPAL includes: uranium processing, biomedical applications, neutron scattering materials, accelerator science, etc., and research excellence has been achieved in several areas, such as: waste conditioning, laser enrichment, high performance materials environmental toxicology.

The Australian Young Generation in Nuclear has recently been created by young scientists from research and industry.

## International co-operation

In a country suffering the dilemma of a non-nuclear-power country with E&T needs numerically smaller but harder to sustain through a national E&T infrastructure, international interaction is becoming increasingly important, as clearly recognised by the UMPNER panel.

The widening and enhancement of international collaboration has allowed improved leverage and further links are being sought. With its current skills and research expertise in many areas, Australia could contribute to international R&D efforts.

Australia is engaged already in various international initiatives, both multilateral, primarily under the IAEA through the participation to Co-ordinated Research Projects, as well as bilaterally, with several individual partners (e.g. with the Korea Atomic Energy Research Institute and with the Department of Energy in the United States).

Existing regional links are also currently established through the IAEA with the Asian Network for Education in Nuclear Technology (ANENT) and through the Forum for Nuclear Co-operation in Asia[1] (FNCA) with the Asian Nuclear Training and Education Programme (ANTEP).

## References

Commonwealth of Australia (2006), *Uranium Mining, Processing and Nuclear Energy – Opportunities for Australia?*", Report to the Prime Minister, Department of the Prime Minister and Cabinet, Australia.

IEAust (2006), Nuclear Engineering Panel of the Institution of Engineers Australia, Submission to UMPNER, September 2006, IEAust, Australia.

NEA (2000), *Nuclear Education and Training: Cause for Concern?* OECD, Paris, France.

1. www.fnca.mext.go.jp/english/panel/e_panel.html.

# Belgium

## Introduction

In Belgium the Education and training (E&T) activities are carried out by academic institutions and the Belgian Nuclear Research Centre (SCK•CEN). The SCK•CEN covers 45% of his turnover directly from a government grant; the rest is from contract works and services.

## Government activities

Due to a series of governmental decisions, the future for nuclear power generation in Belgium is at this moment quite uncertain. A law for the gradual phase out of nuclear energy production was approved in 2003 for the shutdown of NPPs after 40 years of operation. In 2008, however, a new expert body, the GEMIX group, was established by the Belgian government to study the ideal energy mix for Belgium, with a look at multiple nuclear scenarios and a focus on security of supply, competitiveness and protection of the environment and climate. The final report issued by the GEMIX in late 2009, concluded that without the three oldest nuclear power plants, Belgium will face a severe energy shortage by the end of 2015. Based on this, the Belgian government decided to reconsider the 2003 phase-out law and to prolong the operational lifetime of the three oldest nuclear power reactors by ten extra years. Due to the political crisis at the time, however, the parliament never confirmed the government decision, and thus the original phase-out law still remains in place.

The government has also decided to support the MYRRHA project, a flexible fast spectrum research reactor, with EUR 60 million spread over 5 years. Important international projects such as MYRRHA constitute a factor of appeal for young researchers in the nuclear field. Furthermore, the government subsidises colloquia to promote the Belgian Nuclear higher Education Network (BNEN) programme "Master in nuclear engineering" (see below). In 2010 the subsidy was used for the BNEN seminar on Generation IV reactors.

## University activities

In 2001, SCK•CEN and five Belgian universities founded the BNEN (bnen.sckcen.be), with the sponsorship of the Belgian nuclear industries (a sixth university joined during the academic year 2006-2007). BNEN is an example of joint effort to maintain and further develop a high quality programme in nuclear engineering. The intent of the programme is to remodel nuclear education in Belgium, catalysing networks between academia, research centres and public utilities. BNEN has instituted the "Master after Master", obtained from different nuclear programmes merged into a single course for holders of a master degree in engineering. Highly modular, the course is taught in English. Through this programme highly qualified engineers will be prepared for the safe operation of the nuclear power plants, not only in Belgium but also internationally.

**Figure A2.1: Evolution of student numbers in the BNEN programme**

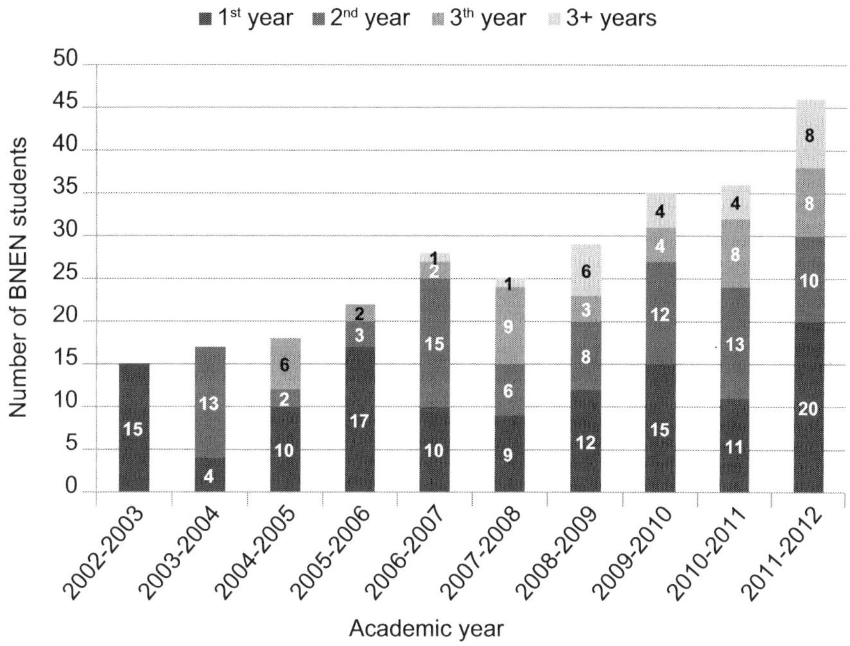


Further master courses of the duration of four years in nuclear technology, medical nuclear techniques and radiochemistry are organised by three Belgian institutes (NEA, 2004).

In 2003, SCK•CEN, XIOS Hogeschool Limburg, *Institut Supérieur Industriel de Bruxelles* together with the *Institut national des radio-éléments* (IRE) joined efforts to start up a radiation protection expert course that gives the qualification of "radiation protection expert", as defined in the Belgian legislation, based on the EU-directive 96/29/Euratom. The programme of 120 hours entails courses on nuclear physics, radiation physics, radiochemistry, applied dosimetry, radiation biology, principles of radiation protection and applied radiation protection (taught in Dutch and French) (NEA, 2004). The programme also includes European and Belgian regulation and legislation (NEA, 2004).

Universities in Belgium have a tradition of informing and recruiting students in any field of study (including the nuclear field), for instance through a "bachelor-day" and the "master-day", when students can liaise with professors and lecturers and learn about the different programmes. In addition, SCK•CEN has also initiated early interactions with potential students. On a monthly basis pupils from the last year of high school have the possibility to visit SCK•CEN and talk with its experts.

## Industry activities

The Belgian nuclear industries support the BNEN programme and actively participate to the shaping and optimisation of its master programme during stakeholder meetings organised on a regular basis. Good collaboration is ongoing between the industry and the research institute SCK•CEN. GDF SUEZ, organises a one-year training for their newly engaged engineers and two weeks of this programme are delivered by SCK•CEN. SCK•CEN also provides customised training programmes for professionals (mainly working in the nuclear industry), mainly in fields like radiation protection, nuclear engineering, decommissioning techniques and nuclear safety, but also in other nuclear topics.

## Research institute activities

Thanks to its vast experience in the field of nuclear science and technology, its innovative research and the availability of large nuclear installations, SCK•CEN is an important partner for education and training projects in Belgium as well as at international level. The centre's know-how and infrastructure are available for education and training purposes. Preserving and extending nuclear knowledge on fundamental and peaceful applications of ionising radiation to serve society is one of the key elements in SCK•CEN's research policy. SCK•CEN co-ordinates and organises training programmes for professionals working with ionising radiation in nuclear technologies, radiation protection, nuclear emergency management and waste management, decommissioning and other topics covered in its research. SCK•CEN's education and training activities are co-ordinated by SCK•CEN's Academy for Nuclear Science and Technology. The Academy forms the centre's own personnel but also trainees from the public and private sectors (nuclear industry, the medical sector and authorities in the field of nuclear applications), contributing as well to the training of Euratom inspectors, ALARA experts and personnel responsible for international transport of radioactive material, etc.

SCK•CEN has strong links with academic institutions. In addition to the joint programmes described above SCK•CEN supports, every year since 1992, PhD candidates or postdoctoral researchers, providing guidance in the preparation of their theses.

**Figure A2.2: Number of post-docs at SCK•CEN**

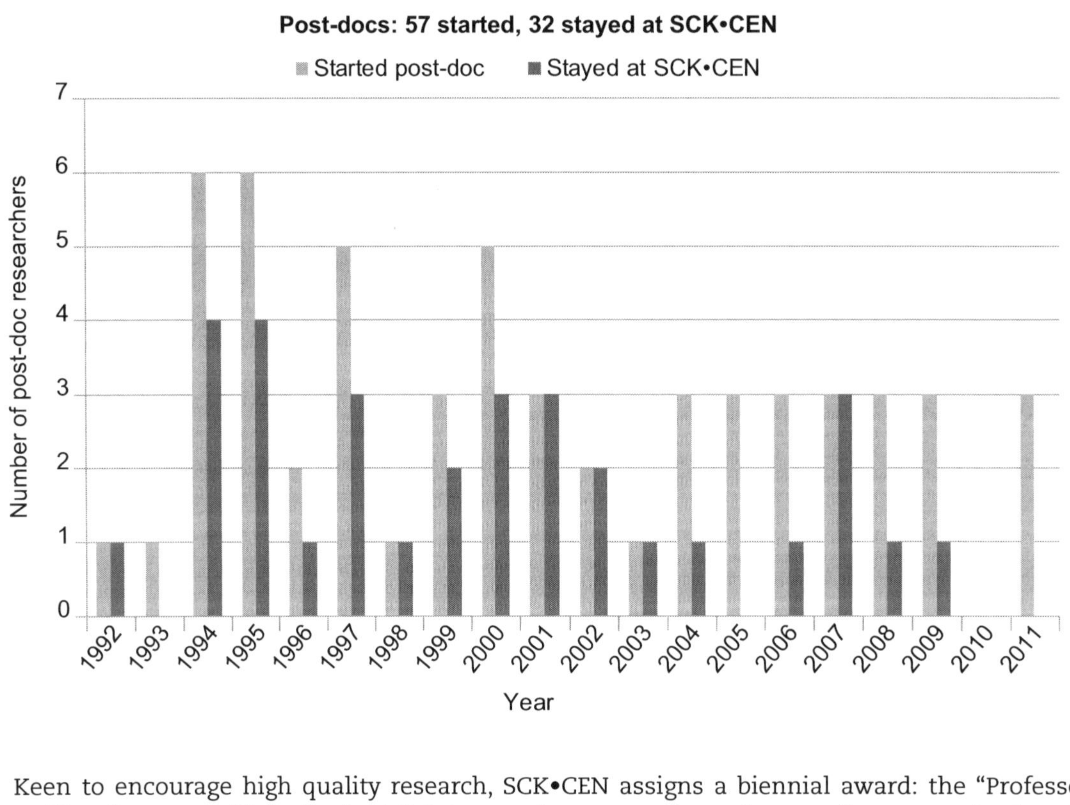


Keen to encourage high quality research, SCK•CEN assigns a biennial award: the "Professor Roger Van Geen award", to the best Belgian nuclear research work, as well as annual prices to the best master theses carried out in its laboratories (NEA, 2004). International students are also hosted by SCK•CEN for internships.

Moreover some SCK•CEN experts have professorship at universities where they teach modules in regular academic programmes.

 NUCLEAR EDUCATION AND TRAINING: FROM CONCERN TO CAPABILITY, ISBN 978-92-64-17637-9, © OECD 2012

## International co-operation

SCK•CEN is an active member in many E&T international networks and programmes. It is the co-ordinator of the European Network on Education and Training in Radiation Protection (ENETRAP). The current project ENETRAP II has the overall objective of developing European high-quality "reference-standards" and good practices for E&T in radiation protection, with the ultimate deliverable of introducing a radiation protection "training passport" as a means to facilitate efficient and transparent European mutual recognition.

SCK•CEN is also part of the steering committee of the European Training and Education in Radiation Protection Foundation (EUTERP) (www.euterp.eu), a European umbrella organisation aiming to harmonise criteria and qualifications for professionals in radiation protection (RP), favouring mutual recognition and facilitating transnational access to vocational E&T infrastructures within the European Union.

SCK•CEN played an important role in the European Nuclear Engineering Network (ENEN) (2002-2004) and its successor project Nuclear European Platform for Training and UNiversity Organisations (NEPTUNO – 2005), whose goals were to safeguard and spread nuclear knowledge and expertise, and to create a European education area in the field of nuclear engineering. ENEN paved the way for the creation of the European Nuclear Education Network Association (ENEN) of which SCK•CEN is an active, central member.

Figure A2.3: **Number of PhDs at SCK•CEN**

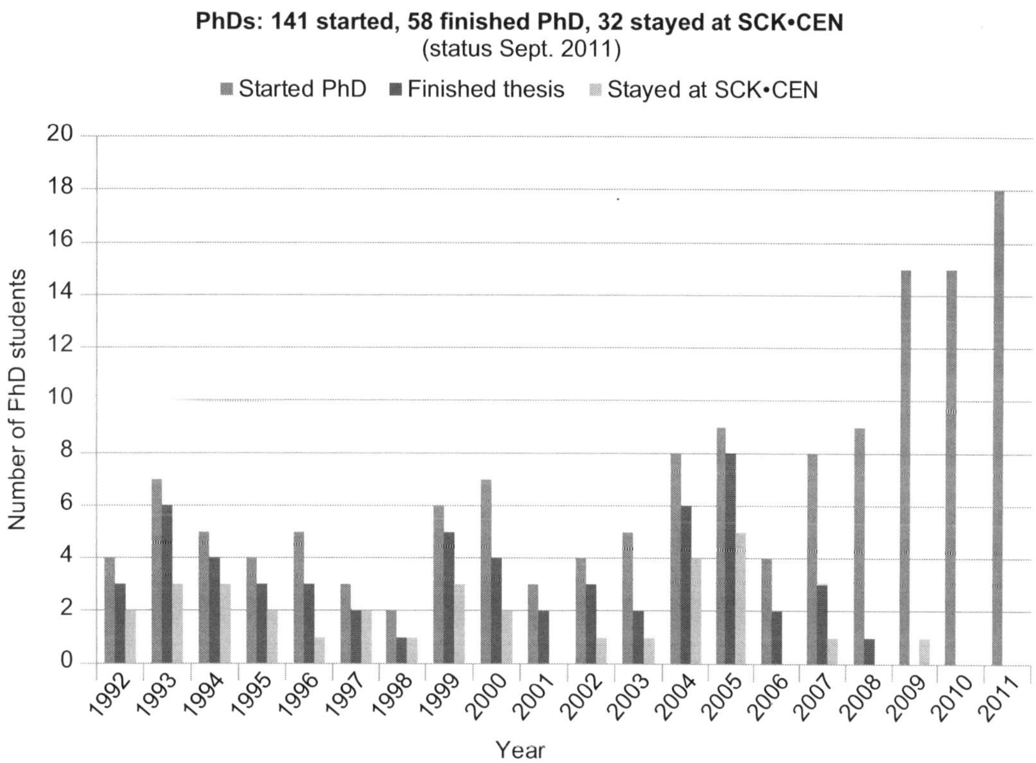


The main objective of the ENEN Association is the preservation and the further development of expertise in the nuclear field through higher education and training, by fostering the co-operation between universities, research organisations, regulatory bodies, industry and any other organisations involved in the application of nuclear science and ionising radiation. ENEN promotes several activities to provide resources and lecturers for training programmes; to establish and develop databases to preserve nuclear knowledge; to assist universities in attracting talented students and recruiting new academic members in nuclear disciplines; and to support high profile projects and research involving students though internships and the development of theses at master and PhD level.

Further, SCK•CEN is involved in several seven FP projects such as ENEN III, ENEN-RU, ECNET and TRASNUSAFE.

Together with several technical universities, SCK•CEN was involved in the ERASMUS intensive programme "Stimulation of Practical Expertise in Radiological and Nuclear Safety" (SPERANSA – 2006-2008). A ten-day practical course was given in Belgium, giving students the opportunity to analyse practical safety aspects of relevant radiological and/or nuclear applications in the nuclear sector, making available, for this purpose, specialised facilities that are normally not accessible to students. A similar programme will be carried out in 2012, focusing on radiation safety and radiation protection.

## Reference

NEA (2004), *Nuclear Competence Building*, OECD, Paris, France.

# Canada

## Introduction

In Canada, energy is the responsibility of the provinces, whereas development, design and (to some extent) construction of nuclear power plants have been largely done by Atomic Energy of Canada Limited (AECL), a federal crown corporation. Each province therefore plans its own energy needs, with the federal government providing the underlying nuclear science and engineering technology.

Human resource planning is, to a large extent, the responsibility of the individual organisations (utility, design, research), although a significant role in development and supply of highly qualified personnel (HQP) has been played since 2002 by the University Network of Excellence in Nuclear Engineering (UNENE). UNENE, a not-for-profit organisation, was founded with the support of the nuclear industry (utilities and design organisations) and the federal government, to co-ordinate nuclear education at the university level in order to meet industry needs.

## Government activities

Most of the current nuclear R&D in Canada is done by Chalk River Laboratories (CRL), which obtains its funding from both the federal government (for more fundamental research) and nuclear utilities (for R&D relevant to station operating and safety needs). CRL has been a major source of HQP over the decades.

Government funding for nuclear education and research in universities is partly through the federal Natural Sciences and Engineering Research Council (NSERC). NSERC supports research projects and therefore the development of qualified graduate students. In the nuclear energy field, NSERC generally matches investments made by the nuclear industry. In addition the provincial governments give a per-student grant to their universities in all faculties, including nuclear engineering.

UNENE is the main educational network in Canada for nuclear power and related activities, comprising 12 universities, nuclear federal agencies and nuclear industrial organisations including operators, designers and the regulator. It was founded to fulfil the following objectives:

- to ensure and enhance a dependable supply of highly qualified and skilled professionals for the Canadian nuclear industry, to meet its current obligations and emerging challenges;
- to create a group of respected, university-based nuclear experts for public, government and industry consultation; and
- to reinvigorate university-based research and development in nuclear engineering and technology, focusing primarily on mid- to longer-term research.

Nuclear Engineering Chairs at Canadian Universities are supported by a combination of industry funding (either directly or through UNENE) and government co-funding.

UNENE currently supports seven Industrial Research Chairs in various universities in areas related to nuclear power. The Chairs in turn generate HQP through their graduate students. UNENE also sponsors several collaborative R&D projects awarded to other researchers at Canadian universities. It also sponsors and co-ordinates a Master of Engineering degree jointly offered by member universities. The course is accredited by the Ontario Council of Graduate Studies. Aimed at people working in the industry, it includes weekend classes, to accommodate students with a full-time job, and synchronous interactive distance education for those at remote sites who might not be able to physically attend the courses (due, for instance to severe weather conditions). In order to deliver a full breadth of nuclear engineering courses, the programme exploits professorial expertise residing at participating universities and draws specialist guest lecturers from UNENE industry members. The programme has graduated 68 students (to 2011), and there are 50 currently enrolled towards an MEng in nuclear engineering.

In 2007-2009 the UNENE investment in nuclear research was instrumental in the successful award of an additional USD 43 million. These funds included a CAD 4.8 million grant from the Ontario Research Fund – Research Excellence programme, to establish "Nuclear Ontario: A University-Based Network Supporting CANDU Nuclear Technology in Ontario"; and CAD 24 million from the Canada Foundation for Innovation and Queen's University. NSERC matched research funding from industry in UNENE and other funding sources. The additional funding has been used to increase the scope of research programmes, build stronger research teams and establish and support nuclear research laboratories and facilities.

## University activities

Beside the UNENE-sponsored programmes, most UNENE member universities have their own research-based graduate courses pertaining to nuclear energy. As of September 2009, the current number of graduate students in the research programmes UNENE-wide is over 130. The number of MSc. and PhD students who graduated during the same period amounted to 26 MScs and 25 PhDs. The University of Ontario Institute of Technology (UOIT) in particular, being located near two of the large multi-unit nuclear power stations in Ontario, has a major undergraduate programme and (since recently) a graduate programme aimed at developing staff for the operating stations.

Both UOIT and McMaster University also offer a Diploma Course in Nuclear Engineering for students who want to improve their knowledge in more specific areas and in a shorter period of time. Undergraduate enrolment in UOIT has been about 250 in nuclear engineering, and 35 in health physics and radiation science.

Still, with a decision on new nuclear build not yet taken in Ontario, convincing undergraduate students that there are careers in the nuclear industry remains a challenge. However the steps toward approval of new nuclear build at Darlington are progressing: on 25 August 2011, the report of the Joint Review Panel for the proposed Darlington New Nuclear Project was released, and concluded that the Darlington New Nuclear Project will not result in any significant adverse environmental effects given available mitigations.

## Industry activities

With respect to industry, all the major organisations run training programmes for in-house staff, generally of good quality but of course not for academic credit. They have also donated much of their training material to UNENE as a supplemental resource for its professors and students. UNENE constitutes a unique industry-university alliance. To help achieving UNENE's goals, the industry is investing significant funds in selected universities and is contributing in-kind to enable universities to acquire and retain the highest quality of teaching and research professoriate. The industry is also assisting the universities in developing relevant research programmes, attracting bright students, and educating them to pursue safe and efficient use of nuclear technology. The universities secure additional funds from NSERC and elsewhere, to match investments made by the nuclear industry. This is a win-win approach and represents the biggest achievement with industrial involvement.

A website (CANTEACH) has been set up as a publicly-accessible repository of all open nuclear information related to education generated by the industry. It is also used as a resource by UNENE.

A recent restructuring within the nuclear industry may also improve educational initiatives. The commercial arm of AECL at Sheridan Park, Mississauga, including its CANDU reactor line, has been sold to SNC Lavalin and will become CANDU Energy Inc. The AECL research arm, mainly at Chalk River Laboratories, will in effect become more of a national nuclear laboratory, with a much broadened mandate. This mandate is still under development, but is expected to include much more co-operation with universities, including making CRL facilities more available to university students and researchers, hosting students on-site as part of their degree work, etc.

## International co-operation

UNENE has collaboration agreements with the World Nuclear University (WNU) and European Nuclear Educational Network (ENEN) and is pursuing meaningful contact with OECD/NEA and similar organisations internationally to promote sharing of best practices, professor and student exchange, distance education, collaborative university-based R&D, sharing course material, and mutual recognition of courses/degrees.

## Reference

NEA (2000), *Nuclear Education and Training: Cause for Concern?* OECD, Paris, France.

# Finland

## Introduction

Finland has four operating units, another unit under construction in Olikuoto (Olikuoto-3 EPR) and a decision in principle has been granted by the Parliament in favour of new NPPs. However, in terms of manpower, to support existing and new plants the situation appears susceptible to future deficiencies, as most experts are soon due to retire and only two professorships are in place in the entire country. Since late 2002 there has been increased awareness of education needs in nuclear safety which led to the establishment, in 2003, of national nuclear courses (YK), resulting from the collaboration of the whole nuclear community in Finland: government, universities research institutes and nuclear authorities. YK courses have significantly helped boosting the number of students (basic courses are now attended by approximately 100-150 students per year, masters by 10-20 students per year) and professionals with academic degree, have nearly doubled since 2000 (to about 1 000 people). It transpires that the nuclear field has been lately of greater appeal to the young generation, whilst interest to open up new education programmes has risen.

Tight connections between the academia, industry, research institutes and authorities are pursued, even if industry is not currently engaged in helping academia funding professorships.

## Government activities

The Ministry of Trade and Industry published in 2000 a report on *Maintaining Nuclear Competence in Finland* and in 2001, 2005 and 2008, energy strategies have been released by the government. The strategies cover climate and energy policy measures in great detail up to 2020, providing a brief outlook for the period thereafter, up to 2050.

The Ministry of Employment and the Economy has taken actions to promote capacity building in the nuclear sector, for instance driving the establishment of the Finnish Nuclear Education Network (FINNEN) and sustaining the national research programme as well as basic training courses on nuclear safety.

Nuclear research in Finland is well funded, with EUR 47 million allocated in 2007, primarily in waste management (61.2%) and reactor safety (28.4%). Specifically, a volume of funding of EUR 7 million was allocated in 2009 to the Finnish Public Research Programme on Nuclear Power Plant Safety (SAFIR 2010, SAFIR 2014) with 31 projects developed in 8 distinct streams of research (ensuring competence in different areas of nuclear safety and maintaining a strong framework for international collaboration). Nuclear utilities have, however, the biggest share in financing, in line with changes of relevant legislation (in early 2004) (NEA, 2004).

## University activities

Nuclear engineering and reactor physics is taught in three academic units: Lappeenranta (LUT), Helsinki Universities of Technology (TKK) and the Laboratory of Radiochemistry at Helsinki University; whereas nuclear energy related topics (like nuclear physics, radiochemistry, material sciences and construction, power engineering, automation, geology) are taught in several universities. Academic studies are often conducted in tight connection with other nuclear stakeholders, the industry, research institutes and authorities, where students can prepare their theses. Furthermore, summer training periods in industries are compulsory.

In Finland there are only two professorships in the nuclear energy area (including fission and fusion). Nine lecturers take part to FINNEN programmes, offering nine courses at the TKK, and nine courses at the LUT. In 2007-2008 a capacity of 15 students at each institution has been reached (EC, 2009).

## Industry activities

Industry has continuously been engaged in providing training for employees. Since 2009, FinNuclear has started organising and co-ordinating all-around training, education and networking for the Finnish Suppliers Group members. It should be noted, however that the majority of the AREVA contingent working in Finland is outsourced and hence educated abroad.

## Research institute activities

Finnish nuclear energy research has been decentralised into several research units and groups, which operate at different state research institutes, universities, utilities and consulting companies. The most important research institutes and universities taking part in nuclear research are the Technical Research Centre of Finland (VTT), the Geological Survey of Finland, the University of Helsinki, the Lappeenranta University of Technology, the Helsinki University of Technology (HUT), the Finnish Meteorological Institute and the Radiation and Nuclear Safety Authority (STUK). As the national authority of radiation issues, STUK has the laboratories for radiation physics and radiochemistry necessary for monitoring environmental radioactivity (NEA, 2004).

A knowledge management project is ongoing at STUK, with the intent of promoting transfer of knowledge from experienced staff to newcomers. Notably, this approach is being adopted since 2006 for the update of the regulatory guidelines, where working groups led by experienced staff include younger people who can learn firsthand from the experts.

## International co-operation

The universities of LUT and TKK joined the ENEN in 2003 and were also among the founding members of the "World Nuclear University" WNU aimed for global collaboration in mobility and education (NEA, 2004).

The construction of Olikuoto-3 is an example of international industrial collaboration. This brings about issues on the languages used, with the technology coming from France, English generally used as vehicular language, and the operating language being Finnish (manuals and technical documents will have to be translated in Finnish).

## References

EC (2009) *Nuclear Safety in a Situation of Fading Nuclear Experience*, European Commission, May, Brussels, Belgium.

NEA (2004), *Nuclear Competence Building*, OECD, Paris, France.

# France

## Introduction

In its continuing use of nuclear power, France faces numerous challenges, including the development of future generations of NPP, the decommissioning of those reaching their end of life, the operation and maintenance of the existing fleet, the waste management as well as the research and development for future systems (EUR 1 billion have recently been allocated by the government to nuclear research). Efforts to address these challenges must be in recognition and conformity to international requirements, with the additional need to continually update approaches and skills. French offer in nuclear education and training has been well sustained during this last decade and further boosted in recent years and months. However, strain deriving from the expanding nuclear programme as well as the massive retirement of French nuclear employees expected in the forthcoming years, call for the recruitment and training of thousands of scientists and engineers each year both in France and in its partner or customer countries, making E&T in nuclear energy domains an absolute priority.

Over the next ten years, about 13 000 engineers with master of science or PhD degrees, and 10 000 science technicians and operators with bachelor of science degrees will have to be recruited for French domestic and international nuclear power activities. The main employers will be EDF, AREVA, GDF SUEZ, national agencies such as ANDRA, suppliers, sub-contractors, and R&D agencies such as the *Commissariat à l'énergie atomique et aux énergies alternatives* (CEA) and the technical safety organisation, *Institut de radioprotection et de sûreté nucléaire* (IRSN).

In order to satisfy these needs whilst maintaining and sharing a well established culture of safety, security awareness, non-proliferation and environmental protection, a number of education and training programmes have been recently promoted, with the involvement of the industry and nuclear research organisations and under the co-ordination and auspices of the government. These are also aimed at educating the public, policy makers, opinion leaders and, in general all nuclear stakeholders.

Nuclear-energy industrial and R&D organisations have become involved in initial education programmes through their experts. Industrial companies such as AREVA and EDF, and national agencies such as ANDRA,[2] have provided grants to endow chairs in various schools.

CEA *Institut national des sciences et techniques nucléaires* (INSTN) (National Institute for Nuclear Science and Technology) plays an important role in this field through its establishments located in Saclay, Cherbourg, Cadarache and Marcoule. This organisation developed nuclear skills several decades ago and has recently enlarged its programmes including also courses in English.

France has made a commitment to support countries that are ready to create the human, institutional, and technical conditions required to establish a civilian nuclear energy programme that meets all the requirements of safety, security, non-proliferation and environmental protection for present and future generations. In response to the need for competence-building in nuclear energy production, France now offers training opportunities in both French and English education programmes, through the co-ordination of the International Institute for Nuclear Energy (I2EN) in conjunction with *Agence française du nucléaire international* (AFNI). AFNI was created within CEA in

2. www.andra.fr.

2008 to develop government to government partnerships with countries willing to take advantage of French nuclear competence.

## Government activities

The government has commissioned a study to assess needs in high-level nuclear education in terms of specific skills required, the available offer from the education system and potential deficit (OPIIEC, 2008). Released in early 2008, the report gave estimates of HR needs and provided recommendations to universities and engineering schools, already delivering courses in nuclear related fields, for a greater co-ordination of their efforts towards a significant expansion of the educational offer.

To this end, the *Comité de coordination des formations aux sciences et techniques nucléaires* was set up in 2008 by the French Minister for Research and Higher Education, renamed *Conseil des formations pour l'énergie nucléaire* (CFEN) in February 2010.The principal goal of the council is to serve as interface between industrial actors, the government and academic and public institutions and to examine education and training needs, student demographics in different courses and, in general, to assess the education offer and its adequacy. This committee advises the Office of Higher Education on the need to open new academic curricula. Chaired by the High Commissioner for Atomic Energy, CFEN includes members who are representatives of governmental authorities in education, research and industry, academic institutions (universities and engineering schools), principal industrial actors (ANDRA, AREVA, EDF, GDF SUEZ) and subcontractors and the main nuclear R&D public institutions (the French Atomic Energy Commission, CEA and the French Technical Safety Organisation, IRSN).

Close co-operation among these members has resulted in the creation of new curricula and a threefold increase in nuclear graduates within a three-year period, with a total of about 450 B.S., 900 M.S., and 100 PhD graduates in nuclear engineering expected in July 2010, and more than 1 000 M.S. in July 2011.

The International Institute for Nuclear Energy was set up in September 2010. It co-ordinates the international recruitment of students with its academic partners, and promotes the French offer for education and training in partner countries. With the support of the training capacities, tools and experience of French nuclear industry, R&D and academic education resources I2EN is also able to create dedicated programmes on demand, for countries choosing bilateral co-operation including assistance in building specific academic capacity as well as internships in France (see also below). I2EN will also organise dedicated seminars and workshops. Finally, I2EN acts as a technical support for CFEN through its large partnership with academic institutions.

During the International Conference on Access to Civil Nuclear Energy, held on 8 March 2010 at OECD, the President of the French Republic announced the creation of I2EN, to constitute a gateway to international applications of French nuclear science and technology education and to vocational training for foreign engineers, to support the promotion and labelling by CFEN of the French education programmes and to facilitate their access to students, co-ordinate recruitment and promote "nuclear jobs". I2EN is also intended to develop networks and partnerships worldwide, including through the establishment of a "centre of excellence for sustainable nuclear energy" (largely open to new comers), in order to build a strong culture of safety and security and to provide a "think tank" on the main challenges associated with nuclear energy.

## University activities

Presently more than 35 engineering schools and universities all over the country offer nuclear related curricula at a master level (and some at bachelor level). Most of the main universities and engineering schools that provide nuclear-engineering-related education programmes or more specialised courses (e.g. in materials, chemistry and safety) are located in the Paris area, in the Southeast (Grenoble, Saint-Etienne, Montpellier) and West of France (Caen, Nantes) and some in the centre (Bourges, Limoges). These universities offer comprehensive nuclear and nuclear-related engineering programmes, with a capacity for the year 2010-2011 of more than 1 000 students for a master's degree.

Nuclear-energy industrials and R&D organisations collaborate and sustain university education programmes. Some industries have also provided grants to endow chairs in various schools.

### International Master's Degree in Nuclear Energy Science[3]

In September 2009, in the Paris area, engineering schools (Paris Institute of Technology – ParisTech; and *École centrale de Paris* – Supélec), in conjunction with the University of Paris at Orsay (Paris Sud 11) and the INSTN, created an international two-year master-level programme in nuclear energy. The programme also receives the support of industrial enterprises (AREVA, EDF, GDF SUEZ). The curriculum, including five distinct majors, covers all aspects of nuclear energy activity and opens numerous opportunities for employment in the nuclear energy industry or in R&D agencies. The first year of the programme (M1) is devoted to basic courses and the second year (M2) includes five majors: nuclear engineering, nuclear plant design, operations, fuel cycle (engineering or radiochemistry), and decommissioning and waste management. The experimental sessions and training are carried out with EDF simulators. Visits to nuclear sites and a master's thesis (20 weeks) complement the courses. All courses are delivered in English, with the exception of a compulsory course in French language and culture. The programme has a capacity of about 200 students per year, with a majority of foreign students. Admission is open to high-potential international students with a bachelor's degree. Direct admission into the second year of the programme is possible for qualified students.

### International Master's Degree in MAterials science for NUclear Engineering (MANUEN)[4]

In close co-operation with EDF and CEA-INSTN, the Grenoble Institute of Technology (Grenoble-INP) offers since 2007 a master degree course in "materials science for nuclear engineering". This 300-hour course awards a degree suitable for both industry and R&D and it is open to French and foreign students after physics or chemistry M1 level or equivalent, and to engineers (for further professional training). It addresses metallurgical and physico-chemical aspects of the ageing of nuclear fuel under irradiation and materials for reactors and components, and covers topics on safety and economics.

### Master's Degree in "Sustainable Nuclear Energy and Waste Management"

The first year (M1) of a new two-year master programme open to foreigners started in September 2010, in the frame of the *École des Mines de Nantes* (EMN) curricula, with 2 specialities covering reactor physics and operation, as well as waste management in the second year (M2). In 2012, ENSI-Caen, an engineering school in Normandy will implement the nuclear science and applications master. Numerous courses will be delivered jointly for these two masters.

## Industry activities

In France, the industry is highly engaged with training as well as education programmes, funding chairs in schools and universities.

AREVA[5] has recently undertaken ambitious training programmes to satisfy high and diverse recruitment needs, including the development of training centres worldwide in partnerships with important international academic institutions. In 2009, AREVA set up a large training centre in Aix-en-Provence (France). Solutions for nuclear training and the enhancement of all nuclear related skills are provided by AREVA to its partners, customers and suppliers, as well as other stakeholders:

3. www.master-nuclear-energy.fr.
4. http://phelma.grenoble-inp.fr.
5. www.areva.com.

government authorities, nuclear groups, electric utilities and fuel cycle operators, both in France and in the rest of the world. Courses cover all stages of nuclear programmes, focusing not only on scientific and technical subjects on the fuel cycle, reactor design and construction, but also on project management, with specific programmes on nuclear facility operation. These are always based on the best safety level, the experience and know-how developed by the group for its own training requirements. Industrial training is delivered by AREVA in a dozen training centres in France, Germany and United States. Around 500 courses are currently offered, with 100 trainers and several thousand students every year. All teaching methods are used including e-learning, classroom sessions, simulator training and study trips with site tours and also some specific internship. AREVA is also able to set up and manage turnkey training centres.

AREVA together with Axpo AG, EnBW, E.ON Kernkraft GmbH, URENCO Limited and Vattenfall AB have signed an agreement to create the European Nuclear Energy Leadership Academy (ENELA),[6] which originates from an initiative of the European Nuclear Energy Forum (ENEF). The academy offers two training programmes. The first one, destined to young graduates from different backgrounds (engineering, natural sciences, law, economics, social sciences...) with no professional experience, allows them to acquire skills in nuclear management. The second programme trains experienced professionals and senior managers to improve their managerial skills. Finally ENELA will also serve as a think-tank and organise meetings to bring together representatives from the nuclear industry, the political world, the media and civil society. Both courses will provide technical and non-technical training that are mandatory for future middle and top managers.

### EDF[7]

EDF has always developed and maintained strong internal vocational training processes for its personnel, particularly reactor operators, who must undergo both initial qualification training and periodic training. The organisation offers about 1.5 million hours of training per year worldwide, with over 650 different operation or maintenance courses and the support of about 700 trainers, including teachers from engineering schools and universities, in France and abroad. Part of these courses is taught in English. EDF has strongly promoted the international masters mentioned above. In 2008, it allocated EUR 4 million to set up the *Fondation européenne pour les énergies de demain* in collaboration with the *Institut de France* to fund education and research in clean energies by financing high education institutions and projects and by providing grants to students.

### GDF SUEZ[8] *(Belgium and France)*

The Nuclear Trainee Programme for junior employees run by GDF SUEZ combines courses and on-the-job training, with individual coaching by experienced company managers. This programme promotes the development of junior engineers (about 100 per year) into nuclear generalists, also favouring their networking within the group. The topics taught range from nuclear fundamentals to safety, including PWR operation, fuel cycle, waste, and decommissioning. A programme for Majors is also implemented for experienced engineers who lack a nuclear-energy education.

## Research institute activities

*The Commissariat à l'énergie atomique et aux énergies alternatives* (CEA)[9] welcomes numerous students in its laboratories offering opportunities to develop PhD theses on numerous R&D topics, in tight co-operation with the industry. Very open to receiving international students, CEA aims to attract more of them in the future.

6. www.enela.eu.
7. www.edf.fr.
8. www.gdfsuez.com.
9. http://www-instn.cea.fr/.

Created in 1956, within the CEA, the National Institute for Nuclear Science and Technology (INSTN) has since provided technicians, engineers and researchers with highly specialised courses in nuclear science and technology, including graduate-level curricula and today it offers a selection of nearly 210 continuing education sessions. These include training for engineers and PhD students in English, on physics and basic operation of light water reactors, decommissioning and waste management, fast neutron reactors, nuclear materials, etc. To attract top-quality national and international PhD students and researchers, INSTN started the "International School on Advanced Studies in Nuclear Engineering" in 2007, consisting of nine one-week independent doctoral-level courses taught in English. The international school provides a complementary scientific background for doctoral students which saw, in 2008-2009, 130 participants, 20 of which were foreign students. The programme, designed for PhD students, is also open to nuclear-engineering researchers.

INSTN also participates in the "train the teachers and instructors" programme created in 2009 and discussed later.

### *Institut de radioprotection et de sûreté nucléaire*[10]

The IRSN is in charge of the training of medical personnel and other workers exposed to radiation in the workplace. The institute also provides a wide range of advanced training sessions in nuclear safety and regulation, as well as initial training in radiation protection. Some of these training sessions lead to qualifications that are recognised throughout France.

Together with other European Technical Safety Organisation (TSOs) IRSN has created a professional training institute in the field of nuclear safety (the European Nuclear Safety and Tutoring Institute – ENSTTI), to design new training programmes which aim, in the first instance, at establishing a common culture in nuclear risk assessment amongst regulators and TSOs within Europe. A further goal of the institute is to contribute to bridging the gaps in expertise and research in the field of safety for the development of civilian nuclear energy programmes throughout the world, in partnership with the European Union and the IAEA.

## International co-operation

Bilateral co-operation has been recently initiated between France and other countries [e.g. China, with the launch of the Franco-Chinese Institute of Nuclear Energy (IFCEN) in Zuhai (Guangdong), Japan, with the institution of a diploma with Tokyo University, Poland, Jordan, etc.] and partnerships amongst French nuclear energy stakeholders have been further strengthened.

The INSTN co-operates with several international organisations, in particular with the IAEA and the European Commission. In close collaboration with the EC and especially within the ENEN framework the INSTN has promoted many national and international partnerships, contributing to the higher nuclear education in Europe.

### *Training of teachers and instructors*

The presence in France of all kind of nuclear activities and facilities represents a unique opportunity to "train the trainers". Through the collaboration of the major French nuclear players, a new course for trainers, instructors and scholars has been implemented, in close co-operation with the interested countries and specifically tailored to their needs and local education system.

10. www.irsn.fr.

 NUCLEAR EDUCATION AND TRAINING: FROM CONCERN TO CAPABILITY, ISBN 978-92-64-17637-9, © OECD 2012

The training, offered in English, covers a broad range of topics and activities, including visits to major French nuclear sites, possible internships, advanced courses in nuclear engineering, hands-on practice, soft skills such as communication and public acceptance. In addition, assistance in designing local training programmes can also be provided.

## Reference

OPIIEC (2008), *Étude sur l'évolution des métiers de l'ingénierie nucléaire,* Observatoire paritaire des métiers de l'informatique, de l'ingénierie, des études et du conseil, Paris, France.

# Germany

## Introduction

Germany is an interesting case as nuclear has not featured as an option in the government strategic energy planning already for some years. Inevitably this has had a strong impact on nuclear E&T. Despite such adverse political conditions however, good effort has still been registered in Germany in the last ten years.

## Government activities

Limited support has been provided by the government for nuclear E&T and few programmes have been kept active, with emphasis principally on nuclear safety and waste management. The German government promoted however the establishment of networks for nuclear research and education, being actively involved.

## University activities

In recent years, in spite of the unfavourable political situation and in contrast to previous and recent forecasts (as shown in Figure A2.4), the number of professors in nuclear education has seen a considerable rise. Projections from previous surveys (2000, 2002 and 2004) are reported in the bar chart and compared with actual numbers. The figure reveals that, in 2010, there were 20 professors in nuclear education (down from 22 in the early 1990s and up from 10 in 2004); a much healthier figure than what trends derived from the survey in 2000 and 2002/2004 had predicted (according to which, in 2010, respectively 10 and 5 nuclear professorships were expected to remain active).

**Figure A2.4: Projections of number of professors in nuclear education in Germany**

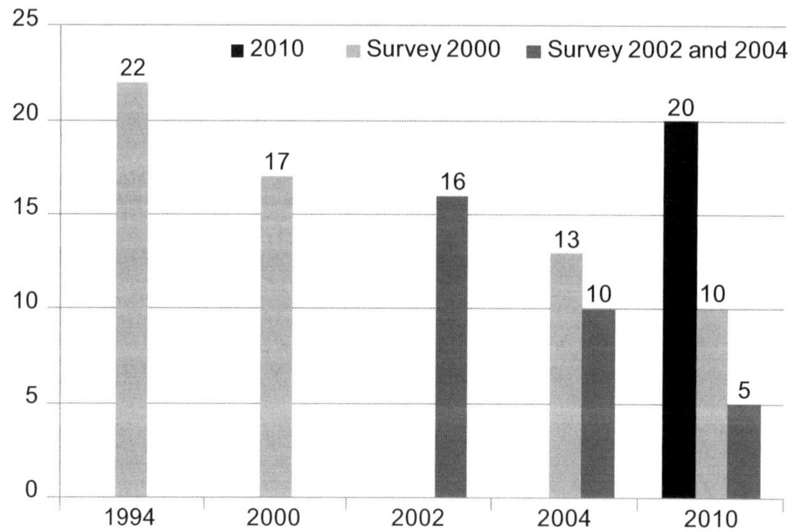




NUCLEAR EDUCATION AND TRAINING: FROM CONCERN TO CAPABILITY, ISBN 978-92-64-17637-9, © OECD 2012

Several universities have been working on the establishment of master courses in nuclear engineering. An increase in the number of both undergraduate and graduate students in nuclear engineering has been observed. Education, especially at PhD level, has been enhanced through the development of attractive research topics and international collaboration projects. Effort has been made to achieve first contact with students as early as possible through several initiatives such as "mentor projects" or a prospective real time NPP simulation platform for research and education, planned by some universities to attract more students to nuclear disciplines.

## Industry activities

In the last decade, significant effort has also come from the industry, with various nuclear education associations being established and collaboration with educational and research institutions, in particular at PhD level, being strengthened (e.g. by financing PhD research work).

AREVA has recently founded the nuclear professional school, in co-operation with KIT, to provide high level nuclear education to engineers and scientists, including AREVA employees and students (including PhDs) at KIT. Experts of KIT and AREVA NP provide a combination of compact courses, with practical research work at institutes of KIT and trainee courses at AREVA NP. In addition, nuclear industries such as EnBW, AREVA, have also sponsored professorships at German universities, significantly contributing to sustain and enhance nuclear education in Germany.

## Networks

Various nuclear educational networks and associations have been established over the last decade through the combined effort of research centres, the nuclear industry, universities and the government. The "Alliance for Competence in Nuclear Technology" (in German: *Kompetenzverbund Kerntechnik*) was established in 2000. In the following years, other associations were also formed, oriented either towards regional needs or related to specific technical areas (e.g. the Eastern Competence Centre; the South-western Nuclear Research and Education Alliance; the Western Nuclear Forum; the Competence Alliance of Radiation Research; and the Repository Research Group). The main goals of these networks are: the identification of future nuclear HR needs and the evaluation of education and training capacity; the enhanced collaboration between universities and international networks; the co-ordination of R&D projects on nuclear safety and waste management; the promotion of young nuclear scientists and engineers (including lecturers for education courses); the provision of student internship, to develop theses at master or doctoral level at facilities near their homes; the participation in further developments of international nuclear standards.

## International co-operation

Collaboration in nuclear E&T between German academic and research institutions with international partners has been ongoing. Several German universities, research centres and industries are members of ENEN. A trilateral partnership in nuclear education (at master level), has been formed between French, German and Swedish institutions.[11] In addition, efforts have been oriented to establish collaboration with non-EU countries; for example KIT is working on an exchange programme for nuclear students with Chinese universities.

11. In the framework of KIC InnoEnergy: http://eit.europa.eu/kics1/kic-innoenergy.html.

# Italy

## Introduction

Italy is quite a unique case in the nuclear international arena. Having been the 4th nuclear power in the world at the beginning of 1960s, Italy has had a moratorium of nuclear lasting some 20 years (since 1987) which makes the country the only G8 member without operating nuclear power plants. Recently, steps were taken to re-enter the nuclear sector, with the objective of building at least four NPPs by 2030. However, following the accident at Fukushima Daiichi these plans were abandoned.

During these years of moratorium, however, skills and capabilities have, to a large extent, been kept alive through the participation of several Italian organisations in European projects and initiatives and as a result of having to deal with the legacy of the previously operating power plants, which has required skills in areas like safety, waste management and decommissioning.

Industries such as Ansaldo and institutions such as the *Ente per le Nuove Tecnologie, l'Energia e l'Ambiente* (ENEA) as well as the Inter-University Consortium for Nuclear Technology (CIRTEN) have been involved in many international programmes, doing research, project management, engineering, procurement and construction activities.

In addition, public bodies have continued their work of monitoring safety and security in all the non energy (medical, industrial) nuclear applications. Seven universities now offer master degrees in nuclear engineering, with approximately 100 graduates per year. A significant challenge is the replacement of professors at these universities.

## Government activities

In the context of an incipient restart of a nuclear programme, various agreements and partnerships had recently been established. In 2006, a formal agreement was set up between the Ministry of Energy, ENEA and universities in order to assess, in collaboration with industries and utilities, future needs for nuclear E&T. Financial resources were provided to reinforce present nuclear courses and to start new ones and funds were made available by the government (2009-2011) to ENEA to start a comprehensive review of the skills needed to resource the national nuclear programme.

## University activities

Historically seven universities have kept offering nuclear courses at different levels (Bologna, Milano, Palermo, Pavia, Pisa, Roma and Torino), with approximately 100 students enrolled each year.

These "nuclear universities" founded the CIRTEN Consortium in 1994 with the aim of promoting nuclear scientific and technological research and co-ordinating the development of nuclear knowledge and collaboration with national and international research institutions and industries.

Recently two new master courses have started at the Universities of Bologna (2008) and Genoa (2010), the latter partially funded by the EU. A new international master degree in nuclear safety and security has been launched at the University of Pisa in 2010, with the collaborative effort of industry, research centres and institutions (e.g. Ansaldo Nucleare, CIRTEN, ITER Consult, etc.).

Links with European programmes such as the European Master of Science in Nuclear Engineering (EMSNE) have been established (notably by the University of Pisa) and are considered key.

Collaboration between universities and the industry has been strengthened, and opportunities are offered to students to develop their theses, undertake training and internships, visit plants and benefit from grants.

## Industry activities

Albeit strongly penalised by the moratorium, Italian nuclear industry has kept active. ANSALDO, the main Italian nuclear manufacturer, provides engineering and construction services for plant completion, plant upgrading, component replacement and plant life extension. ANSALDO Nucleare has been operating mainly abroad in joint ventures with international groups, such as Westinghouse, AECL (for the construction of five CANDU reactors in Cernavoda, Romania) (NEA, 2004) and Toshiba-Westinghouse with a recent important job order for the construction of the first AP1000 in China.

In 2005, ENEL, the main Italian electricity utility, and *Electricité de France* signed a memorandum of understanding that gave ENEL a 12.5% share (some 200 MWe) of the new Flamanville-3 EPR nuclear reactor (1 650 MWe) in France, and potentially another 1 000 MWe from the next five such units.

The industry is generally engaged in providing training "in the field" to personnel and to re-create nuclear competences. ENEL has a sustained group of employees deployed and seconded internationally in the construction and operation of NPPs in Easter Europe and France; and so does ANSALDO. Electronic and component industries such as D'Appolonia are engaged in preparing people for a prompt deployment of qualified manufactures for nuclear applications.

The master degree is aimed at graduates in engineering and in technical and scientific subjects who wish to gain specialised skills in nuclear plant implementation. The master degree course supplies basic multidisciplinary skills in the nuclear sector. Its executive format (on average three days a week over 18 months) has been devised for professional people and qualification awarded to participants is recognised by academia.

Partnerships are being established with dedicated companies (such as Apave Nuclear Power Services) for training, consulting and qualifying Italian engineers and technicians.

## Research institute activities

Overall, about 200 people are dedicated to research activities in the nuclear field and the importance of raising the level of commitment in such activities was recognised as key for the potential development of a new nuclear programme.

The main scientific organisation in Italy is the CNR (Italian National Research Council). This public organisation of great relevance in the field of scientific and technological research dates back to 1923.The research performed in the nuclear field by CNR focuses mainly on physics, chemistry and related topics. On average 10-15 grants are awarded every year by CNR on the nuclear field. Theoretical research in nuclear is also performed by the *Istituto Nazionale di Fisica Nucleare* (INFN) and some more applied research activities are still carried out at the facilities of Pavia, equipped with research reactors (LENA 250 kW).

The leading agency for applied nuclear research in nuclear energy is ENEA through its "Energy Research Centres" of Bologna (ENEA/RB3 100We), Roma-Casaccia (ENEA/TRIGA 1MW and ENEA/TAPIRO 5 kW) and Brasimone (Fast liquid metal reactors for Generation IV). Several research reactors are also operating in various universities, including AGN Constanza (operating at the University of Palermo since 1960), LENA Triga II (250 kW, operating at the University of Pavia since 1965) and a number of subcritical assemblies.

## International co-operation

Bilateral agreements have been recently established to help the development of a Human Resource Plan through the exchange and use of knowledge, people and infrastructures; notably between Italy and France and Italy and the United States, at an intergovernmental level, and between ENEL and EDF, AREVA and CIRTEN, ENEA and CEA/IRSN.

ENEA, universities and industries play an active role in international research co-operation working with IAEA, NEA, EURATOM, GNEP and Generation IV. Multiple domains are covered, such as:

- safety for existing and advanced/innovative reactors (SARNET2);
- simulation and modelling (NURISP);
- the development of innovative systems (GEN IV, IRIS, ELSY, RAPHAEL, CDT);
- waste management (EUROPART, EUROTRANS; ACSEPT); and
- radiation protection.

## Reference

NEA (2004), *Nuclear Competence Building*, OECD, Paris, France.

# Japan

## Introduction

Until the accident at Fukushima Daiichi, nuclear power plants produced about 30% of total electricity in Japan. Nuclear human resources development has been and is still an essential issue for all nuclear-related organisations in Japan. Additionally, the number of developing countries that plan to introduce nuclear power is increasing and Japan is expected to provide technological assistance to such countries, including training for engineers.

Recent trends of declining student enrolment and nuclear workforce registered up to 2005 seem to have reverted, with the numbers now on the increase. On the other hand, retirement of senior engineers and researchers at nuclear facilities has raised the issue of technical knowledge transfer from old to young generations; whereas the decreasing numbers of faculty members and relevant facilities at universities has also posed serious challenges in sustaining programmes in nuclear subjects. Therefore, the need to invest in nuclear E&T through the collaboration of all relevant stakeholders has been increasingly pressing.

A number of positive steps have characterised HRD in Japan over the last ten years, including government policies as well as academic programmes and collaboration, sustained R&D activities and the involvement of industries.

In 2005, a senior network activity in the Atomic Energy Society of Japan was started by some retired experts, who, on a voluntary basis, take the initiative to talk directly to the young generation, mostly students doing university courses in fields not related to nuclear. The frequent meetings organised (more than 30 between 2005 and 2009), seemed to have been successful in making young people appreciate various aspects of nuclear energy and its applications.

After Fukushima Daiichi accident, no remarkable changes have been observed in the number of students who major in nuclear-related subjects at universities (in mid-2011), but most sectors including nuclear industry, research organisations, and the academic society fear that young generations would change their mind and leave nuclear fields. The trend could emerge in the student number enrolled in 2012.

## Government activities

In 2007, the Nuclear Human Resources Development (HRD) Council was established through the collaboration of the government, industrial and academic entities and R&D organisations to address mid and long-term requirements for the development of nuclear human resources. During the years 2007-2009, the council has conducted several investigations, such as quantitative analyses, visions, roadmaps as well as international aspects related to nuclear human resources. The council issued two middle-term reports (in 2008 and 2009) and in 2010 a final report (CNHRD, 2010), which includes ten proposals for nuclear HRD in Japan and recommendations to all stakeholders, encouraging specific nuclear HRD activities.

The government has also provided important financial support to universities and industrial organisations to strengthen their education and training systems. In 2007, the Ministry of Economy, Trading and Industry (METI) and the Ministry of Education, Culture, Sports, Science and Technology (MEXT) sponsored a programme to sustain universities and colleges in their education plans on nuclear engineering and science, with more than 30 institutions involved in the programme every year (35 universities and colleges in 2010).

Some regional activities in relation to nuclear HRD are also being promoted by local governments in conjunction with nuclear organisations. For instance, the Prefecture of Fukui, which counts 13 nuclear power plants and a fast breeder reactor (Monju), has initiated a plan to create a regional hub for R&D activities in various fields of science and technology as well as nuclear HRD, to provide training and education facilities for Asian and Japanese apprentices. This is a joint project which results from the co-operation of local governments, utility companies, universities, manufacturers and the Japan Atomic Energy Agency (JAEA).

The Japan Nuclear Human Resource Development Network (JN-HRD Net) has been recently initiated by the government. In autumn 2010, this nationwide project set up the Japan Nuclear HRD Network consisting of academic institutions, industries, public bodies and R&D organisations, a national framework of organisations in the field of nuclear HRD for education and training of students, young researchers and engineers in Japan. With 62 participating organisations as of summer 2011, the network is aimed at co-ordinating initiatives of member organisations and conducting inter-sector activities in order to address the important proposals of the Nuclear HRD Council, with JAEA and the Japan Atomic Industrial Forum Inc. (JAIF) playing a key role.

## University activities

Some universities in Japan are developing and introducing new nuclear education programmes for graduated students. In 2005, the University of Tokyo has established the Professional School of Nuclear Engineering, which awards qualifications such as "nuclear reactor supervisor" and "nuclear fuel handling supervisor" as well as the Professional Master Degree. A comprehensive curriculum is taught over one year and a total 16 students per year attend the school, mostly sent by nuclear organisations, such as utilities, nuclear facility manufacturers, as well as regulatory bodies. The school is operated in co-operation with JAEA, which dispatches more than 70 experts (researchers and engineers) as visiting professors or lecturers every year, with more than 90% of experimental exercises conducted at JAEA research facilities (including accelerators, neutron irradiation facilities, etc., as well as various types of reactors). At the University of Tokyo, a course on "nuclear energy sociology" has also been started, covering three major "social-related" subjects: nuclear law and regulation, nuclear non-proliferation and the harmonisation of society and nuclear technology.

Collaboration between different academic institutions is also well established. Lectures and practical exercises on nuclear engineering are conducted in collaboration with industries (utilities and manufacturers) as well as JAEA at universities willing to run nuclear related courses but lacking professional staff. The Japan Nuclear Education Network (JNEN) is a good example of this type of collaboration. Established in 2007 by three universities and JAEA (now extended to six participating universities), JNEN is a unique remote-education platform which uses internet-base systems so that students can access to lectures provided by professors in other universities or taught remotely. Technical exercises are also provided for the students by JAEA using its facilities.

Under the Global Nuclear Human Resources Development Initiative, a new framework of university network activities, called the University Union, has been recently formed. Tokyo Institute of Technology, leading university of the union, and 14 universities of Japan are now conducting new education programmes for their students. The union has also started a joint international activity, sending Japanese professors to provide a one-week seminar to students and young researchers in nuclear-developing countries.

## Industry activities

As reported above, numerous initiatives in nuclear HRD in Japan have seen the involvement of the industry, with fruitful collaboration and networks being established with academic institutions and governmental bodies.

In general, individual facilities perform "on-the-job training" for their own staff, ensuring the transfer of technical knowledge from the elder to younger personnel. Most utility companies conduct systematic programmes and with dedicated equipment, such as large scale nuclear power plant operation simulators for the training of their personnel. In addition, strict collaboration is often sought with universities and R&D organisations, such as JAEA, for the training of personnel under Japan Nuclear HRD network.

## Research institute activities

JAEA is the largest organisation for R&D on nuclear technology in Japan. It was established by the merge of Japan Atomic Energy Research Institute (JAERI) and Japan Nuclear Cycle Development Institute (JNC) in 2005. Through its Nuclear Technology and Education Centre (NuTEC – recently renamed the "Nuclear Human Resource Development Center": NuHRDeC), originally founded in 1975, JAEA conducts a wide variety of training courses for engineers and scientists, seminars for government and local government officers and educational activities for the public. JAEA collaborates closely with universities and professional schools. It holds co-operative agreements with 20 academic institutions, dispatching experts (researchers and engineers) as lecturers and inviting students from these universities for research experiments in its laboratories. As reported above, JAEA, in collaboration with the University of Tokyo, founded the Professional School of Nuclear Engineering in 2005 and has been recently helping connecting several universities through JNEN and its Internet-based platform.

Figure A2.5: **Number of trainees at NuHRDeC domestic courses**

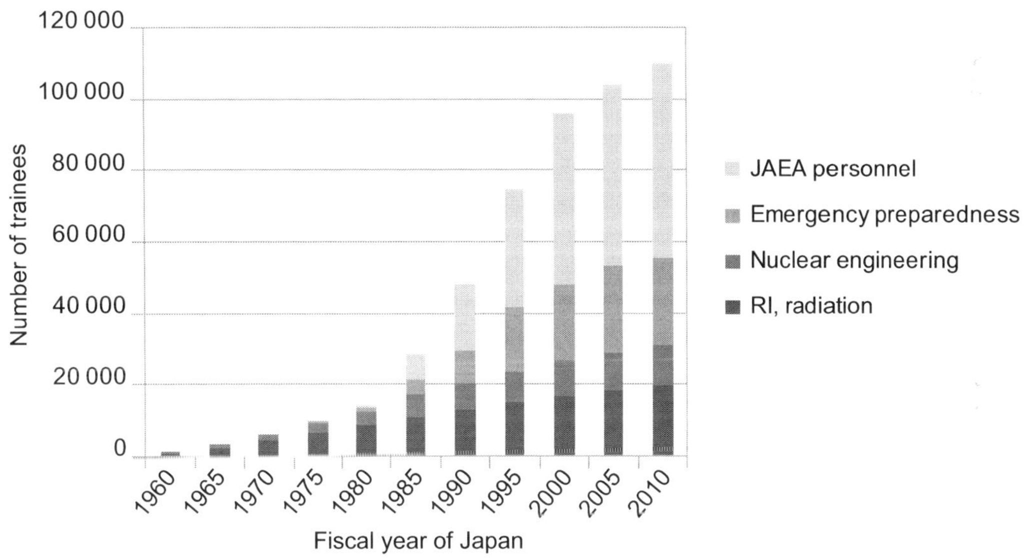


## International co-operation

Japanese universities promote the collaboration with foreign institutes or international organisations dispatching young students, researchers and engineers to international training courses and internships. Some Japanese academic institutions actively co-operate with IAEA, ANENT, WNU and ENEN.

JAEA is engaged in many international E&T activities. The Instructor Training Course (ITC) and Follow-up Training Course (FTC) are international training programmes originally started in 1996 for two countries, Indonesia and Thailand. At present, they have been extended to 7 countries, including Bangladesh, Kazakhstan, Malaysia, Philippines and Vietnam. Through these programmes, trainees from participating countries are invited in Japan to attend courses by NuHRDeC, which in turn sends experts for training and lecturing activities in these countries. JAEA co-operates with the Forum for Nuclear Cooperation in Asia (FNCA) which is a Japan-led co-operation framework for the peaceful use of nuclear technology. The FNCA organises workshop on HRD every year with the participation of Australia, Bangladesh, China, Indonesia, Korea, Malaysia, Philippines, Thailand and Vietnam and it is creating a database for nuclear HRD. JAEA also contributes to the ANSN (Asian Nuclear Safety Network) activities by providing technical information on nuclear safety through an Internet-accessible database. In co-operation with IAEA, JAEA organises Safeguards Training Course every year since 1996. Furthermore, In Autumn 2010, Japan joined IAEA-ANENT (Asian Network for Education in Nuclear Technology) and further co-operation activities with IAEA are anticipated.

## Situation of nuclear HRD in Japan after the Fukushima Daiichi accident

The accident at Fukushima Daiichi nuclear power plants left no other choice for the Japanese government than commencing a review of its nuclear energy policy. In the report issued at IAEA Ministerial Conference, the importance of human resource development, especially in the fields of nuclear safety and emergency preparedness was expressed. Recently, Japan Nuclear HRD Network announced a message to the network member organisations, a guideline for future nuclear HRD activities with some important task items to be addressed triggered by the Fukushima Daiichi accident. Through these activities, the network and its member organisations are aiming to contribute to the strengthening of nuclear safety in Japan. Some of such new HRD activities had already started under financial support of the government.

## Reference

CNHRD (2010), *Report of the Council of Nuclear HRD*, Council on Nuclear Human Resources Development, Tokyo, Japan (*in Japanese*).

# Korea (Republic of)

## Introduction

Korea has an expanding nuclear programme, with 21 nuclear power plants in operation and 18 more either under construction or planning domestically. Recently Korea has also embarked in export contracts for the construction of NPPs in the United Arab Emirates (2009) and of a research reactor in Jordan.

The Korean nuclear manpower pool is still sound, with the increase of the number of NPPs. The nuclear R&D activities has been stabilised after the Legal Nuclear R&D Fund was established, raising nearly USD 1 per MWh of electricity generated. With these ambitious plans the Korean nuclear industry will have to double in size at least, which makes nuclear HRD a very crucial issue.

Ageing of nuclear experts in research institutes is of some concern, even if not severe, worsened by the governmental policy to reduce the size of the public sector. Universities have suffered from the dearth of talented students, as the new generation tends to avoid science and engineering topics. Manpower shortages are experienced in all areas. This increasing awareness has led the government Ministry of Education, Science and Technology (MEST) to expand resources for manpower development since 2002.

Due to the limitations in human resources, joint research initiatives among industries, universities and/or research organisations have been particularly beneficial in Korea, allowing the development of original and self-reliant indigenous technologies.

Although restructuring of the Korean electricity market is ongoing since 1999, the major nuclear related organisations are still under state control. The main nuclear industries are Korea Hydro & Nuclear Power (KHNP), KEPCO Nuclear Fuel Company (KNFC), KEPCO Engineering and Construction (KEPCO E&C), KEPCO Plant Service (KPS) and KHNP Central Research Institute (KHNP CRI), which are under the jurisdiction of the Ministry of Knowledge and Economy (MKE). The main research institute and regulatory expert group are respectively the Korea Atomic Energy Research Institute (KAERI) and the Korea Institute for Nuclear Safety (KINS) that depends from the MEST. In October 2011, a new governmental organisation, Nuclear Safety Commission (NSC), is expected to be established to achieve the independence of the regulatory organisation.

## Government activities

A few policy studies regarding nuclear manpower are being launched by the government.

Because of the high involvement of the state in the nuclear sector, government policy is very important and influential to each aspect of the nuclear industries. Over the years, the Korean government (MEST) has adopted a very systematic approach in addressing HRD, with the Comprehensive Nuclear Energy Promotion Plan (CNEPP). The CNEPP, originally formulated in 1995 by the Ministry of Science and Technology (MOST), now MEST, is developed on a quinquennal basis (currently by the MEST) to define high level directions and objectives as well as more detailed planning for budget and investment, covering infrastructure and manpower.

In 2002, prompted by a decline of student enrolment and the number of nuclear experts, the Korean government, through the MOST, sponsored a study on the domestic nuclear manpower status. In the study, the OECD/NEA report published in 2000 was cited to emphasise the worldwide situation of nuclear manpower, education and training. Since then, the government has been expanding its nuclear manpower development programme.

In these last ten years, the Korean government has greatly increased educational support. Beside the Brain Korea 21st century (BK21) programme, started in 1999, by the Ministry of Education, the Ministry of Knowledge and Economy also established manpower development programmes for industries and universities related to electric industries. Whilst previously university funding was restricted to basic and applied science and engineering research, the recent expansion of programmes in support of universities allows diversified research, also suited for educational purposes (NEA, 2004).

More specifically in relation to nuclear E&T, the MEST has provided grants to support research of undergraduate students. Under the programme, started in 2003 (see also NEA, 2004), about 70 to 80 students have been selected annually with individual research grants of about USD 7 000.

The Nuclear Technology Undergraduate Student Society (NtUss), also sponsored by MEST, has provided its members with a research camp, has organised visits to research institutes and nuclear facilities, and lectures and conferences. All such activities are designed to give the young people an overall picture and some experience of the nuclear industry, while promoting networking (NEA, 2004).

The MEST has provided nuclear E&T grants of USD 0.1 million to each of the eight nuclear engineering departments in Korea.

The MEST and the MKE are currently formulating and re-designing their nuclear human resources development programmes recognising that it is one of the three major issues that should be resolved urgently.

## University activities

Student enrolment in nuclear engineering has suffered the general trend experienced in all technical subjects in Korean universities. The Korean Nuclear Engineering Department Heads Organization (K-NEDHO), formed in 2001, discussed extensively the issue, playing a prime role in heightening the government awareness on the problem and triggering several governmental initiatives (as described above).

University research grants are on the increase. Longstanding internship programmes for students exist in the research institutes and industrial organisations, with internship often leading to employments. Graduate students participate in R&D projects run by KAERI and KINS. Through such programmes the next generation of researchers is formed, while enhancing the co-ordination between research institutes and universities.

## Industry activities

The KHNP has expanded its own manpower development programme to a mid- and long-term training and education programme for its employees. The courses (about 150), consisting of internal and external training programmes at domestic and foreign institutes, cover different nuclear and nuclear-related topics, including also management and leadership courses. Some 500 open courses are also provided by KHNP for the industry and the public. Web-based lecture and training programmes have also been developed to help remote training.

KINS training programmes are very comprehensive, encompassing in-house programmes, international co-operation initiatives, such as the "International Nuclear Safety Master Degree Programme" as well as courses for the public.

KEPCO has recently (December 2009) received the government approval to launch the KEPCO International Nuclear Graduate School (K-INGS). Due to open in March of 2012, the school represents the first KEPCO education programme completely devoted to nuclear energy; it will be located next to the Kori nuclear power plant, giving its students easy access to on-the-job training and practical learning experiences. With a funding close to KOR 58 billion (USD 49.6 million),

K-INGS plans to accept 200 students per year, offering 2-year programmes with specialised courses in nuclear energy planning, operation, and maintenance.

The KHNP together with the MKE has established and sponsored the Korean Nuclear Energy Foundation (KNEF) for the dissemination of objective scientific knowledge about the peaceful use of nuclear energy to enhance public understanding and awareness as well as to educate future generations on nuclear energy. Under this initiative scholarships are offered and projects for the dissemination of information in the field are co-ordinated in the vicinity of nuclear power plants (NEA, 2004). KNEF holds nuclear facility visits for undergraduate students, with approximately one hundred students visiting NPPs under operation or construction every year (NEA, 2004).

## Research institute activities

The age distribution in research institutes is higher than what reported for the industry, although bulk retirement is not expected for a while. Nevertheless, research institutes are gradually raising their recruitment rates in order to replace the retiring researchers.

KAERI has kept providing an extensive in-house E&T programme, including both fundamental and advanced courses, for its own members as well as for industry personnel and university students. Both, practical and managerial courses, including research reactor training for undergraduate students in nuclear engineering are delivered, whilst a series of Web-based education and training programmes has also been set up (NEA, 2004).

KINS established in 2004 the Nuclear Safety School to foster world-class nuclear safety regulators by operating effective systematic expert education programmes and to contribute to an upgrading of Korea's position in the international community by actively sharing international nuclear safety information. In co-operation with the Korea Advanced Institute of Science and technology (KAIST), KINS also runs the unique "KINS-KAIST International Nuclear Safety Master's Degree Programme".

## International co-operation

KAERI is very active in promoting international co-operation through multilateral and bilateral programmes in education, as well as research and development. It organises educational programmes and courses for the IAEA and the Word Nuclear University. It co-operates with the Asia Network of Higher Education on Nuclear Technology. ANENT was established in 2004 to assist countries in the Asian region in nuclear education, knowledge management, and related research and training. KAERI is developing the ANENT Web-portal and Web-based education and training programmes together with the IAEA and its member states in the region. KAERI is also providing technical support to developing countries, transferring to them its method and programmes for manpower development. Since 1998, it has organised training courses for developing countries under the IAEA/KOICA programme.

At the academic level, Korean universities have established international collaborations in nuclear education. For example, since 2003, sponsored by the MEST, students from six Korean universities have been sent to visit Kyoto university research reactor and have two weeks of training overseas.

KHNP is actively engaged in international co-operations with IAEA, Institute of Nuclear Power Operations (INPO), WANO, etc. Recently, driven by the expectation of increased exports of Korean NPPs, the MKE and the affiliated organisations are planning to expand their international co-operation activities and have established the "Nuclear Export Association" to support the government towards enhanced international collaboration.

## Reference

NEA (2004), *Nuclear Competence Building*, OECD, Paris, France.

# Spain

## Introduction

The Spanish government has not established a strategic energy planning in relation to nuclear energy. The decommissioning of Zorita NPP as well as the decision to reduced the period of license for the life extension of Garoña NPP only to three years, instead of ten, have conveyed a negative message to the new generation of students and even professionals. Despite this, all nuclear stakeholders in Spain have maintained high levels of nuclear E&T, allowing an influx of students which has been adequate to meet human resource demand for domestic needs. Although in Spain public opinion on nuclear energy is one of the worst of the EU, the young generation has been receptive in getting involved in education training programmes in the nuclear field, partly enthused by the recent perspective of a global renaissance.

The Spanish Nuclear Regulatory Body (CSN) has dedicated funds to promote and enhance activities on R&D in nuclear safety and radiation protection and to support master courses in nuclear science and technology. CSN has also recently created and sponsored three chairs in two universities.

Formal support by the Spanish government to nuclear energy is deemed key in order to stimulate more interest amongst young people, and to spur E&T.

## Government activities

The government has maintained nuclear educational programmes and staff at universities. In addition it has promoted the creation of large nuclear infrastructures such as ALBA, the synchrotron accelerator in Catalonia, the SNS-Bilbao and the Neutron Source Installations in the Basque country, as well as the establishment of new research programmes such as TECHNOFUSION and CONSOLIDER, run by universities and the National Research Centre on Energy (CIEMAT).

## University activities

Universities have been very active in maintaining and adapting their syllabus in nuclear education (e.g. through the implementation of the Bologna system), offering scholar grants, ensuring good interaction with potential students through regular seminars, collaborating with the industry.

Nuclear Engineering and Master Programmes are active in three universities and CIEMAT, with some courses taught in English. Courses on nuclear subjects are also taught in other universities and, although not always well attended, some of these courses are compulsory when undertaking master studies in energy.

In most countries, the accreditation of a master course of nuclear engineering follows the same rules as the accreditation of any other master course in engineering. However, in Spain, the good quality of the Spanish nuclear education has been certified by the Spanish National Accreditation Agency (ANECA). The *Universidad Politécnica de Madrid* (UPM) has received the ANECA Quality Award for its Masters in Nuclear Science and Technology, which allows inviting foreign professors under government support. Very recently it has also been accredited by ABET.

In the effort to attract more students several activities have been promoted: the Open University (UNED) in Madrid has implemented distance learning and some other universities are offering also new attractive advanced courses (including transmutation, material science, advanced computer codes, nuclear fusion technology, nuclear science applied in industry and medical applications) in addition to basic subjects (as nuclear physics, nuclear technology, nuclear safety and radiation protection).

The Politechnical University of Madrid is well integrated in European and international frameworks and has established collaboration with industry and research centres. However it is deemed that further participation in fission and fusion international research programmes and the involvement of industry in research and training may still improve the situation.

Very recently the Polytechnical University of Catalonia has launched a new Master in Nuclear Technology in collaboration with one of the Spanish utilities (ENDESA).

## Research institute activities

Research institutes, notably CIEMAT and the Institute of Nuclear Fusion at UPM, have been very active in high profile research programmes, but also in education and training activities, in collaboration with universities and international research centres.

The National Technology Platform for Nuclear Fission Energy R&D CEIDEN was created in 2007 to co-ordinate the needs and efforts of the Spanish R&D in the field of fission nuclear technology. Within this framework a one-year Master in Nuclear Technology and Applications (MINA) has been established in 2008 by CIEMAT, with the collaboration of several universities, the support of the nuclear industry and the participation of an increasing number of students from Spain as well as South America.

Nuclear research is also conducted in other research institutes in various universities (such as the Institute of Nuclear Fusion at UPM), also involved with education programmes such as master courses and tutoring and doctoral theses, in collaboration with other national and international institutions (e.g. the Lawrence Livermore National Laboratory, Universities as Nevada, Penn State and others).

The resulting enhanced mobility and the interest of the research topics developed have attracted new students, contributing to sustaining HR needs in the Spanish nuclear sector.

## Industry activities

Spain has a very strong nuclear industry with facilities operating in various segments of the fuel cycle and nuclear related activities (e.g. ENUSA and ENRESA operating in the fuel cycle, ENSA manufacturing heavy components, engineering companies such as *Empresarios Agrupados* and Tecnatom and, of course, utilities operating NPPs) and a very active regulatory body.

Whilst the HR needs for the domestic industry have been satisfied so far, potential future gaps transpire from current projections, caused by impending retirement of experts and the rising needs. New training programmes are being set up, notably by the engineering companies Tecnatom, *Empresarios Agrupados* and CIEMAT.

The Foro of the Nuclear Industry and the Spanish Nuclear Society (SNE) have also played an important role in nuclear E&T. Foro started several years ago disseminating information on the nuclear energy and its advantages in intermediate and high schools, to professors and students. In collaboration with UPM the Foro has organised seminars all over the national territory and it has also promoted summer schools for young university students in collaborations with universities. During the last four years, UPM and Foro have co-organised three Summer Schools inviting Spanish and European professionals and journalists. Amongst the various activities of the SNE, are very good E&T programmes, such as the Basic Course on Nuclear Energy run during the last three years in several universities and institutions, and the provision of grants and prizes to young students.

## International co-operation

Strong networks with other European universities and nuclear research centres have also been established through the participation to international R&D programmes, mainly within the Euratom framework (e.g. ENEN, ENEN-II, ENEN-III, ENETRAP, NEPTUNO, PETRUS, TRANSNUSAFE) and with the WNU.

# Sweden

## Introduction

In Sweden, after the difficult times experienced as a result of the phase-out decision, the nuclear sector has recently seen a significant shift, with the governmental decision in early 2009 to allow the replacement of old reactors.

The Swedish Centre for Nuclear Technology (SKC) was formed during the difficult years by the three nuclear power plants (Forsmark, Oskarshamn, Ringhals), Westinghouse and the Swedish Radiation Safety Authority to ensure that nuclear engineering programmes at the universities were not completely abandoned. SKC ensures national co-ordination, provides base funding for education and research, promotes and co-ordinates joint research projects and attractive educational programmes, which increase the interest to enter nuclear technology among students. It aims at creating strong and internationally recognised research groups within areas which are vital for and unique to nuclear technology.

In Sweden, the nuclear education is now in a very good state, with a healthy and increasing number of students and professors. If maintained, this positive trend could lead, in a few years, to the formation of a class of Swedish nuclear engineers which may even slightly exceed current domestic needs.

## University activities

Different education programmes are active in Swedish universities at various levels, with new academic activities just started or about to start. Different syllabus and course contents are adopted by different universities in their nuclear educational programmes. This is considered positive, as nuclear science and technology are multifaceted fields, and with various professional specialisations (albeit built on a common background) better satisfy the different industry needs.

Until recently Sweden never had a dedicated nuclear engineering programme at bachelor level, but one has started in the autumn 2010 at Uppsala University. A third-year specialisation in nuclear engineering will be added to an existing three-year bachelor course in mechanics engineering to allow students from any technical college or university with a background in mechanical or electrical engineering to complement their knowledge with topics on nuclear technology. Since 2008, the Royal Institute of Technology (KTH) in Stockholm offers an international MSc in nuclear engineering. The programme has attracted 10-15 students per year. Courses are also open to students participating in other programmes, so that an average attendance of about 25 students per course is reached. In the autumn 2009 the Chalmers Institute of Technology, in Gothenburg, has also started a new nuclear engineering MSc. The programme, encompassing in equal shares courses in reactor physics/technology and nuclear chemistry, forms expert knowledge which reflects industrial needs, providing well prepared staff for the nearby Ringhals nuclear power plants.

In the same academic year, Uppsala University has started a nuclear engineering specialisation programme which complements a general engineering programme in energy systems.

Presently, there are about 60 students in Swedish universities, conducting 4-year PhD programmes. This is an approximate number of 15 PhD students enrolled per year, with numbers slightly on the increase. This healthy enrolment has already helped boosting other activities.

Nuclear courses attract a good number of students and the enrolment is increasing with a good proportion of overseas attendance. Foreign students are admitted to all higher Swedish education, and nuclear engineering is no exception. Restrictions apply only to students from countries which have not signed the nuclear non-proliferation treaty (NPT criterion). Often, but not always, teaching is conducted in English. At KTH and Chalmers, about 100 foreign students per year apply to each of the nuclear engineering programmes, both taught in English. Only a small proportion is however accepted (7 foreign students at KTH and 5 at Chalmers in 2009) based on the NPT and other selection criteria aimed at ascertaining the preparation of applicants, as in many cases, the quality of previous exams is difficult to ascertain.

A generation change has been successfully achieved in the university faculties, with an age profile of tenured professors in nuclear power related research and education shifting towards younger ages. This transformation has been possible thanks to the collaboration and support of the SKC and the Swedish Waste Management Company (SKB) that made a historic effort in the 1990s to help young nuclear scientists.

One side effect of the recent academic generation change is a much improved collaboration climate. The traditional Swedish academic system was based on individual careers with lifelong contracts for full professors and very unsecure working conditions for younger staff. The new generation professors have established themselves through entrepreneurial activities, performing research and education for external parties (industry, authorities, the EU and research councils). Thereby, they have accrued greater experience in project management, seeking a collaborative approach. Today these young professors promote collaboration across boundaries, contrary to old practices when individuals often pursued their own careers.

Unfortunately Swedish universities do not have research reactors as the last one was closed a few years ago. Nevertheless universities have collaborations with industries and international academic institutions running research reactors, where students are sent for training.

All the universities have bilateral collaborations with industries and the authority agencies. Typically, the nuclear power plants support the geographically closest university for recruitment purposes.

## Industry activities

The Swedish nuclear industry is presently in a state of re-juvenation. During the coming ten years, due to retirements and to increased needs in HR for new-build, 6 000 new staff are expected to be employed, which in volume corresponds to the entire present industry population. However the capacity for education and research is stronger than it has been in many decades, and the industry demand should be satisfactorily fulfilled. There is also an emerging prospect of establishing, if required, a flow of professionals to Germany.

Industries are involved both as sponsors and as contributors with teachers.

*Kärnkraftsäkerhet och Utbildning AB* (KSU) – Sweden's nuclear training and safety centre – provides training and measures to develop staff skills for the Swedish nuclear power industry, according to their short- and long-term needs (KSU, 2009). Founded in 1972, the company is part of the Vattenfall Group and is jointly owned (in equal shares of 25%) by Barsebäck Kraft AB, Forsmarks Kraftgrupp AB, Oskarshamns Kraftgrupp AB and Ringhals AB. A significant part of the competence of Swedish nuclear power operators and maintenance personnel is delivered and maintained by KSU's training programmes (3 964 course-days were delivered in 2009). KSU trains and assures the competence of operators, maintenance staff and other personnel, both through theoretical studies and through the use of simulators (which reproduce power plant control rooms). Training of maintenance personnel is also carried at the closed Barsebäck nuclear power station, providing an authentic nuclear power plant as the training environment. The company also produces and manages educational material needed for its training activities.

 NUCLEAR EDUCATION AND TRAINING: FROM CONCERN TO CAPABILITY, ISBN 978-92-64-17637-9, © OECD 2012

## Research institute activities

Sweden closed its research reactors a few years ago. The only existing neutron facility is the cyclotron-based neutron source at the Svedberg Laboratory in Uppsala, which is operating at energies far above the reactor-relevant ranges. This facility is nevertheless important for diploma work, etc., but not used in regular course studies.

Uppsala uses the TRIGA reactor in Helsinki for its training exercises. Ferries frequently cross the Baltic Sea and part of the courses are taught onboard at the conference facilities of these ships.

KTH has used several different solutions, depending on the student attendance. Beside Helsinki, Mol in Belgium and the training reactor at Budapest University of Technology and Economics have been used. Discussion is in progress about purchasing a dedicated school reactor. The industrial full-scale reactor simulators are also used for student training.

## International co-operation

Sweden has no longer a technical support organisation (like CEA in France or VTT in Finland). Following the privatisation of the Swedish technical support organisation, a very dynamic situation has developed, with the advent of a large number of consultancy companies. Industry and academia need to have direct contacts and collaboration. For a small country, this has some advantages as maintaining such permanent national structures is often very costly and sometime can lead to stagnation.

A significant drawback is however the lack of a research reactor. Since the cost for such a facility is too high for a small country, it would be advantageous if an EU-based system could be established, with shared facilities and shared costs. A private Swedish initiative in that direction is the recent purchase by Vattenfall of 2% of the Jules Horowitz reactor under construction in Cadarache, France.

As already mentioned, given the high number of new nuclear engineers expected to graduate from Swedish universities in the forthcoming years, there is some discussion in progress for a Swedish-German collaboration programme, to deploy young Swedish nuclear engineers at German nuclear facilities, where they could spend the first years of their career, thus giving a contribution to remedy the more difficult staff situation in Germany.

There are many collaborative initiatives between Swedish universities and other European academic institutions, promoting a good exchange of students. Foreign enrolment is relatively high for diploma courses or internships. For example, Uppsala University and *Université de Caen*, France, have a regular exchange programme by which three French students per year spend three-month internship in Uppsala. Similar programmes are common at all the three universities.

## Reference

KSU (2009), *Operating Experience from Swedish Nuclear Power Plants*, Kärnkraftsäkerhet och Utbildning AB, Sweden.

# Switzerland

## Introduction

Switzerland, although perhaps the smallest country represented, has been having, for a long time, as much as 40% of its electricity generated by nuclear power plants. Although there has been little input from the government in recent years as regards the planning of HR needs for nuclear, the nuclear industry itself has been actively monitoring demand and supply. In this context, it has been collaborating very effectively with universities and the national research institute. The unique synergy between industry, academic institutions and the research centre – certainly facilitated by the small size of the country – has been fundamental for the establishment of the new Master of Science degree in Nuclear Engineering, offered jointly by the two Swiss Federal Institutes of Technology, at Lausanne and Zurich, since 2008.

## Government activities

Since many years, mainly due to political factors, the government's strategic energy planning has been strongly in support of renewable energy and energy conservation, with nuclear taking a "back seat". There has, however, always been indirect support to young students, in that both universities and research centres in the nuclear context are governmental institutions in Switzerland. The recent events in Fukushima Daiichi, however, have had a dramatic effect on the government's nuclear policy. In the wake of this most unfortunate accident, it has been announced that the operating plants will be run till the end of their operating lives and not be replaced, so that nuclear energy is envisioned to be phased out entirely by 2034 (assuming a uniform lifetime of 50 years for all the Swiss plants). The government's announcement has received full parliamentary approval, but the final decision – with the direct democracy that Switzerland is – will lie with the population at large, via a national referendum. In any case, one aspect for which there is unanimity is that nuclear education and research remain important, particularly in the context of issues related to nuclear safety and waste disposal.

## University activities

At the university level, economic pressure has, in recent years, caused a shift of educational programmes away from "classical" fields such as nuclear physics, towards domains which currently appear more attractive to young students (life sciences, nanotechnology, etc.). However, significant positive steps have been taken, for example with the establishment, as mentioned above, of a common degree – the Swiss Master of Science in Nuclear Engineering (Swiss NE Master) – by the two Swiss Federal Institutes of Technology at Lausanne and at Zurich. Although the new degree has resulted largely from self-generated motivation at the academic level, it relies heavily on the excellent collaboration mentioned above between the two universities, the Paul Scherrer Institute (PSI) as national research centre and Swissnuclear, the association of Swiss nuclear utilities. The Swiss NE Master represents a true "quantum jump" for the country in terms of additional commitment towards nuclear education, and to date it has registered good success and very positive experience, with some 15 to 20 national and international students attending each year. Since 2010, with the upgrading of the curriculum from three to four semesters, complete compatibility of the curriculum has been achieved with respect to other nuclear engineering programmes in Europe.

## Industry activities

The industry, apart from its key role in monitoring HR needs for the country, has kept providing high-quality, in-house training of their nuclear power plant staff, as well as support to education at the university level. For example, industry helped setting up the current Chair in Nuclear Energy Systems, when the Swiss Federal Institute of Technology in Zurich decided in 2004 to suppress its Chair in Nuclear Engineering. Continuing education programmes are also organised regularly. The active industrial involvement in the Swiss NE Master includes the provision of lecturers in several courses, as well as industrial internships for the students. Industry has also become conscious of the need to provide objective information on energy and environmental issues to pre-university students, a recent survey having shown that students at this stage of their education are much more open to the notion of nuclear energy as part of a sustainable energy mix than are their teachers.

## Research institute activities and international co-operation

PSI, the national research institute at which most of the country's nuclear (fission) energy related R&D is conducted, has been very effective in supporting educational needs. Thus, most of the PhD research in the nuclear field is carried out, not at universities, but at PSI. This has been occurring in the framework of exemplary collaborations with the Swiss Federal Institutes of Technology and the industry, which finances nearly 50% of the R&D activities of PSI's Nuclear Energy and Safety department. A part of the financial support is separately earmarked for PhD students and young scientists. Along with the earlier mentioned example of the joint Nuclear Engineering Master, this collaboration provides ample evidence that the desired co-ordination of efforts has indeed been happening quite effectively in Switzerland, with considerable progress also at the European level, largely through the participation in European Nuclear Education Network (ENEN) activities.

# United kingdom

## Introduction

After a long period of industry decline, with no new station commissioned since 1995, in 2007 the UK government published its White Paper *The Role of Nuclear Power in a Low Carbon Economy*. This generated a significant change in policy development, inter alia the creation of the Office for Nuclear Development and the roll-out of the regulatory process for new build (including generic design assessment and strategic site assessment). No limits have been set to the extent of new build, on the basis that there would be no public subsidy. The scene was therefore set for an integrated HR planning process to emerge.

To sustain the ongoing decommissioning programme (which accounts for approximately GBR 2 billion a year) along with the new build programme, impending nuclear workforce needs in the United Kingdom are estimated to be very sizeable; and, given the high rate of retirement in the forthcoming years, a substantial demand for new recruits is expected. Looking ahead to 2025 some 8 500 people are expected to leave the UK industry due to retirement, corresponding to approximately one third of the current nuclear-specific workforce (WNN, 2011). The profile acts most harshly on the higher skilled and more experienced parts of the workforce, where, up to 70% of current employees are expected to retire by 2025 (Cogent, 2009) Meanwhile, projections by the academy indicate that UK employers could hire about 1 500 new staff each year to fill nuclear-qualified roles (WNN, 2011).

## Government activities

Over the last decade, the government has commissioned various important assessments on the UK nuclear industries. Already around about 2003, as one of the outcomes of the major "Study on Nuclear and Radiological Skills"[12] conducted in 2002 by the Department of Trade and Industry (now Department of Business, Innovation and Skills), the Cogent Sector Skills Council was established to facilitate a direct demand-led link between government, industry and E&T providers. Cogent Sector Skills Council covers several industries, all safety-critical, as well as hi-tech and of strategic importance, including the nuclear industry. Cogent Sector Skills Council is an employer-led organisation but regulators were involved at the outset of its programme.

In 2004, Cogent Sector Skills Council set up a Nuclear Employers Steering Group covering all aspects of workforce planning of the nuclear sector in the United Kingdom (i.e. fuel processing, power generation, decommissioning and defence). The key role of Cogent has been to undertake an in-depth analysis on recent new build labour market, assessing the shape of the workforce in nuclear industry, identifying gaps, growth and the need for training and qualifications; a very engaging task culminating in four "Renaissance" reports:[13]

*Power People: The Civil Nuclear Workforce 2009-2025*, September 2009;

*Next Generation: Skills for New Build Nuclear*, March 2010;

*Assurance: Skills for Nuclear Defence;*

*Illuminations: Future Skills for Nuclear.*

12. www.berr.gov.uk/files/file23311.pdf.
13. www.cogent-ssc.com/research/nuclearresearch.php.

*Power People* provides a comprehensive UK skills panorama of the civil industry today, encompassing the full cycle of operations and bringing into focus future skills on an horizon spanning to 2025. Building on this first report, *Next Generation* identifies the likely demand for skills in support to the nuclear industry for a specified scenario. In particular, a programme is hypothesised which foresees the deployment, by approximately 2025, of 12 PWR units to generate up to 16 GWe. While this is a realistic albeit ambitious scenario, the methodology developed may be applied to other possible circumstances. The report also defines specific skill sets which, due to deficiency in the capacity or capability of their delivery chain and in absence of mitigating measures, could impact the timely accomplishment of the programme. A Nuclear Energy Skills Alliance steering group has been set up to oversee implementation of the recommendations of the *Next Generation* report and to ensure that strategic and critical skills solutions are managed for the emerging new build nuclear sector. The fourth of the series, *Future Skills* for the nuclear industry will capture the preparation for new build activities and long-term planning for decommissioning.

In addition, Cogent has recently published the *Nuclear Skills Oracle 2010* report, which provides a snapshot of the industry labour market from a sizable cross section of employers (200 companies). The *Nuclear Skills Oracle* will supply reliable sector wide data for the development of trend Labour Market Intelligence on an annual basis, providing also a benchmark for individual companies.

Further, a risk matrix of key skills and critical pathways has been compiled and is intended to be extended towards a greater quantification. Currently, large categories have been identified embracing various roles, with more detailed data gathered for the industry only. With respect to construction, for example, a semi-quantitative assessment has already been undertaken, providing some further insight, although, at this stage, this is only preliminary. For a selected number of jobs, role profiles are provided and include a typical job description, key processes, competencies and knowledge needed, as well as pay conditions, entry requirements and applicable industry standards. In addition, with the *Standards and Qualifications Prospectus*,[14] Cogent has listed all the standards and qualifications of relevance to the nuclear industry. In the prospectus, *Nuclear Job Contexts*, families of nuclear industry standard jobs have been developed through a very in-depth appraisal undertaken by Cogent in consultation with the nuclear industry. Thousands of jobs were considered and condensed down into families, which proved to be a very hard task. Through this top-down process Cogent will work their way through in gradually filling up a detailed job cartography, with a defined number of roles to be covered every year. Each job context sets out the competencies, qualifications and training standards that will provide a route to securing skills across each of the above areas.

Cogent is developing a suite of employer-led qualifications that underpin its competency-based Job Contexts. It has recently elaborated a roadmap to higher level skills for the science-based industries represented by the Sector Skills Council, through "technically higher".[15]

The government provides, indirectly, a significant part of teaching and research funds to universities. Despite recession-driven retrenchment, it has committed to fund 10 000 ring-fenced new places at universities for science, technology, engineering and mathematics provision.

With the support of the government and nuclear industry, the "Nuclear Graduates Scheme" has been set up,[16] hosted by the Nuclear Decommissioning Authority (NDA). This is a highly selective nuclear graduate programme, aimed at attracting the best graduate talents to the sector with placement opportunities in the top companies. The scheme entails: two years with four secondments, 480 hours of dedicated training, 10% voluntary time, two dedicated mentors and a dedicated sponsor.

14. www.cogent-ssc.com/Publications/Cogent_Qualification_Prospectus_Nuclear.pdf.
15. www.cogent-ssc.com/Higher_level_skills/HE_Strategy.php.
16. www.nda.gov.uk/news/skills-strategy-launch.cfm.

## University activities

As universities are autonomous, they develop programmes according to their specific missions, in a typically demand-driven fashion. The vast majority of funds (typically amounting to over GBR 20 billion p.a.) come by via teaching or research routes that ultimately originate from government sources.

The prospect of new build has raised the awareness of opportunities to prospective students. However it is important to distinguish between a small but important niche demand for nuclear courses and the large demand from the sector in new build for supply of good science and engineering graduates and technical staff. Craft and technical levels are just as important as the higher engineering roles. On this front universities are providing more nuclear undergraduate modules and working with technical colleges, sometime franchising courses. In several universities (such as Liverpool, Surrey, Birmingham and Manchester) specialist masters are devoted to continue professional development for those in employment in the nuclear sector. Some of these are long-standing courses and, overall, attract some 70-90 recruits per year. In addition, with the Working Higher Project, Cogent is supporting the development and roll-out of modular, work-based foundation degrees.[17] The National Skills Academy Nuclear in conjunction with employers and Cogent is developing a Certificate of Nuclear Professionalism. This post-graduate modular certificate, aimed mainly at new graduates, covers managerial, commercial, project management, communication and technical modules which can be delivered flexibly to satisfy the needs of employers.

The greatest volume demand is for Vocational Qualifications and Cogent is working with industry to develop new courses to cover specific nuclear skills and the National Skills Academy Nuclear is ensuring delivery through their Quality Assured Training Provider Network. This enables verification of training for the Nuclear Skills Passport, facilitating mobility and transferability of skilled personnel.

In terms of encouraging students and providing them with adequate information, universities in the United Kingdom are increasingly giving data on employability of their graduates to prospective applicants. Cogent is developing, with the higher education sector "Graduate Attributes", employability benchmarks statements in the nuclear sector as voluntary standards for the higher education sector to use. Cogent has also set out "Career Pathways", a tool that demonstrates the skills, qualifications, job roles, competencies and career progression for those employed in the nuclear sector.[18]

New nuclear master level courses are also being developed and the UK Nuclear Technology Education Consortium (NTEC) has been created between universities and other institutions to provide postgraduate nuclear education.[19] The structure and content of the programme, which leads to qualifications up to master's level in nuclear science & technology, was established following extensive consultations with the UK nuclear sector, including industry, regulators, NDA, government departments and the Cogent Sector Skills Council. All courses are of modular format and the core content is taught as a one-week module at the relevant institutions. Each module may be taken as a standalone short course for continuing professional development purposes and the option of distance learning is also provided, giving maximum flexibility (e.g. for vocational training of or professionals, or for part-time students). A distance learning platform: WebCT, has also been set up. This web-based Virtual Learning Environment includes handbooks, discussion groups, video clips as well as information on NTEC courses.

## Industry activities

The industry has been committed to the continuous provision of quality training, with new initiatives recently launched. For instance, in 2005, Atkins founded the Nuclear Academy, a training institution for its employees, and in 2008. With the same intention, British Energy, now EDF Energy,

17. www.cogent-ssc.com/Higher_level_skills/Working_higher.php.
18. www.cogent-careers.com/careerpathways.
19. www.ntec.ac.uk/.

 

created the Nuclear Power Academy and Magnox launched the Magnox Graduate Programme. Nuclear industry supports the Cogent National Occupational Standards, National Vocational Qualifications and Foundation Degrees and their delivery via the National Skills Academy for Nuclear.[20] The latter was set up by employers in 2008 to ensure excellence in skills development and provision across the UK nuclear industry. The Skills Academy has established a network of High Quality Providers to ensure that the delivery of programmes is to the highest standards. This employer-led organisation aims to ensure that the UK nuclear industry and its supply chain has the skilled, competent and safe workforce it needs to deal with the current and future UK nuclear programme. One of the principal goals of the National Skill Academy is the development and implementation of the industry wide "Nuclear Skills Passport",[21] recording nationally recognised skills, competencies and training across the industry across the breadth of the skills pyramid. The job contexts are featured on the Skills Passport aligned to the industry agreed training standards, enabling both companies and individuals to carry a detailed training and skills analysis and then plan future skills, training and staffing needs effectively. The Skills Passport will house detailed, current and validated individual learner records enabling and promoting the mobility of staff and the transferability of skills. The industry is making the Skills Passport highly desirable in supply chain tenders so that it can be an effective vehicle for driving up standards across the workforce. Employers have agreed a minimum "bar level" of entry for working in and with the sector which will be recorded and demonstrated on the Skills Passport. This "Triple Bar Standard" includes: basic common induction, basic nuclear industry context, basic nuclear behaviours. The aim of this standard is to ensure that people working in and with the industry understand how and why the nuclear industry is different to other industries and have the right attitudes and behaviours to work safely in this highly regulated industry.

For the nuclear sector, Cogent is providing the learning areas and standards and the National Skills Academy Nuclear is ensuring effective delivery through a network of Higher Education Institutes. This represents a good example of educational networks between universities and the industry to promote education in the nuclear field, with many other industry university consortia, such as the Nuclear Academic Industry Liaison Sub Committee of the Nuclear Institute (NAILs).

In 2009, the British Nuclear Energy Society and the Institution of Nuclear Engineers merged together in the Nuclear Institute (NI), a professional institution and learned society that represents nuclear professionals in the United Kingdom.[22] The NI promotes activities for the advancement of nuclear science, engineering and technology, and more specifically for maintaining high standards of education and professional performance amongst engineers, scientists and others working within the nuclear industry. It also promotes public understanding of nuclear science.

## Research institute activities

With respect to support to R&D, building on existing partnerships with EDF Energy, Rolls-Royce and AWE the new Nuclear Research Centre (NRC), a joint venture between the University of Bristol and the University of Oxford, has officially been opened in late 2011 to help developing a skilled workforce for the UK's nuclear industry. The new centre aims at providing leading edge and innovative research to support the design and safe operation of current and future generations of nuclear systems, including both fundamental research and work on emergent topics (WNN, 2011a).

Further, the National Nuclear Laboratory[23] has been recently established to provide leading nuclear technology services through technical innovation and intellectual support, including: helping to reduce the cost of clean-up and decommissioning, maintaining critical skills, attracting new people to the industry and working with cognate organisations around the world.

Separately, the Nuclear Advanced Manufacturing Research Centre has been created as a joint venture between the universities of Manchester and Sheffield.

20. www.nuclear.nsacademy.co.uk.
21. www.nuclearskillspassport.co.uk.
22. www.nuclearinst.com/ibis/Nuclear%20Institute/Home.
23. www.nnl.co.uk/.

## References

Cogent (2009), *Power People – The Civil Nuclear Workforce 2009-2025*, available at www.cogent-ssc.com/research/Publications/NuclearReportPowerPeople.pdf

WNN (2011), *New Reactors, New Workforce*, available at www.world-nuclear-news.org/NN_New_reactors_new_workforce_0112111.html

WNN (2011a), *UK Prepares for Nuclear New Build*, available at www.world-nuclear-news.org/NN-UK_prepares_for_nuclear_new_build-1011115.html

# United States

## Introduction

The original Nuclear Energy Agency (NEA) report, *Nuclear Education and Training: Cause for Concern?* highlighted many of the difficulties the United States and others were facing with nuclear education and training. At the time, enrolment in nuclear engineering and health physics was flagging, university departments and research and test reactors were closing and the retirement of a large number of nuclear workers loomed on the horizon while the infrastructure needed to train the next generation of nuclear workers withered.

The nuclear science and technology sector in the United States needed a broad array of nuclear workers. Many realised at that time that the United States needed to restock its nuclear education pipelines to ensure that an ample supply of next generation nuclear workers would be available when the majority of the existing workforce retired. A consistent supply of well-trained nuclear tradesmen, technicians, engineers and scientists is critical to ensure the safe and secure operation of the country's commercial power reactors, universities, government research laboratories and other nuclear-related ventures.

A healthy nuclear education infrastructure is the first step to ensuring safety and security at the country's nuclear facilities. For the past decade, the United States has focused on a consolidated effort between the federal government, academia and the industry to solidify the country's nuclear education infrastructure. Emphasis was given to stabilising the number of universities offering nuclear engineering and health physics degrees and developing a new national programme to educate nuclear energy technicians at trade schools and community colleges.

This concentrated effort has been successful. There are 32 ABET accredited programmes in nuclear engineering, nuclear engineering technology and health physics. These programmes no longer have declining enrolments as they did in 2000. They now have more than 2 800 students enrolled (ORISE, 2011). In 2008, there were only four trade schools and community colleges with nuclear energy technician programs (NEI, 2010). There are now 38 of these programmes graduating nearly 500 people a year (NEI, 2012).

This success does not mean that the work is complete. The United States must continue to be diligent in monitoring the state of the nuclear education infrastructure and ensure it receives support from government and industry to remain sustainable.

## Current nuclear science and technology footprint in the United States

It helps to understand the nuclear science and technology footprint in the United States before describing the country's education and training needs. The United States has 104 commercial nuclear power plants that directly employ 60 000 people. An additional 60 000 people are employed at the nation's nuclear vendors, contractors and suppliers. These vendors produce goods and services that maintain the nation's 104 operating reactors by providing fuel, outage services and back-end services to the commercial nuclear fleet.

The US government requires nuclear workers at many different facilities to perform a wide variety of functions. The US Navy maintains 104 nuclear reactors that propel submarines and aircraft carriers. Maintaining this fleet are 40 000 sailors, hundreds of engineers and scientists within the government and hundreds of people working at national laboratories.

The US Nuclear Regulatory Commission (US NRC) is responsible for overseeing the safe and secure operation of the commercial nuclear fleet as well as the country's research reactors. This agency employs nearly 4 000 people spread across their headquarters, four regional offices and field operations.

The US Department of Energy's (DOE) mission is to ensure America's security and prosperity by addressing its energy, environmental and nuclear challenges through transformative science and technology solutions. To fulfill this mission, the DOE manages 16 national laboratories and tens of thousands of people work as scientists, engineers and technicians at these facilities either as direct government employees or as contractors.

Supplementing the national laboratories are facilities with research reactors. There are 31 research reactors operating in the United States (US NRC, 2011). These research reactors are located at universities and both private and public research laboratories.

Supporting this entire nuclear infrastructure are thousands of manufacturing companies. In the United States, the American Society of Mechanical Engineers has certified 383 Nuclear Stamp (N-Stamp) holders (ASME, 2011). This N-Stamp allows them to produce equipment for safety related functions within the nuclear facilities.

Nuclear reactors are not the only nuclear technology utilising across the country. An estimated 16 million nuclear medicine imaging and therapeutic procedures are performed each year in the United States (SNM, 2012). These procedures are conducted at hospitals and clinics by thousands of nuclear medicine professionals.

## Current status of the nuclear workforce in the United States

The United States has numerous nuclear sectors and the status of the nuclear workforce differs between these groups. The US Navy has had a healthy, continuous supply of new recruits going through its workforce. Its workforce distribution includes a large number of younger staff who are working alongside their more experienced co-workers. This recruiting model requires that there be a continuous supply of nuclear knowledgeable engineers and scientists.

In contrast, the nuclear energy industry did not bring many new people into the workforce once new plant construction stopped in the 1980s. This created a workforce that is now heavily dominated by experienced workers approaching retirement. Indeed, 39% of the commercial nuclear energy industry's current workforce will be eligible to retire by 2016 (NEI, 2011). With the large number of employees the industry is projecting to hire, the industry worked together with government and academia to ensure nuclear education pipelines were in place to provide enough new talent to fill vacancies.

## Government activities

Government support has been instrumental to ensuring a healthy nuclear education infrastructure in the United States. But, the government is not the only source of support. Support for nuclear education comes internally from local administration support and externally from the federal government and the nuclear industry. Both external sources need the nuclear education system to be sustained to ensure an adequate supply of graduates is available to fill its vacancies. Federal grant funding has been available to provide support with research, curriculum development, fellowships, scholarships and equipment purchases. Educational institutions have to compete with other institutions to obtain the federal grant funding. Industry tends to focus its funding to provide equipment, scholarships and internships and support for focused research. The external sources are key to internal support where nuclear academic programmes compete will all other programmes for funding.

The Department of Energy's Office of Nuclear Energy (DOE-NE) utilises up to 20% of its research and development funds to fund research at universities. In addition to providing cost-effective research, these funds have the secondary benefit of supporting the work of graduate students so that they can complete research projects as they are completing their graduate degrees. The Department of Energy provided USD 170 million for research at the universities in 2010-2012 (DOE, 2012a).

Even if there is an ample supply of students and professors, nuclear education programmes must find a way to purchase the expensive equipment necessary to provide a top-flight education. DOE-NE helps ensure there is equipment available at the nuclear education institutions by providing infrastructure grants. DOE-NE provided funds for equipment and research reactor upgrades to nuclear education institutions.

The Nuclear Regulatory Commission (NRC) funding provided USD 75 million in 2010-2012. Their grants allowed education institutions the opportunity to diversify their course offerings through curriculum develop grants, new faculty development awards, undergraduate scholarships and graduate fellowships. The NRC also manages a Minority Serving Institution grant that provides financial support to education institutions serving diverse populations. This gives students, who normally would not have access to a nuclear education, the opportunity to learn more about nuclear science and to work in this field.

The Integrated University Program is a joint agency programme aimed at supporting nuclear education (IUP, 2009). The DOE-NE and the NRC both provide grant opportunities to universities, colleges and trade schools. The National Nuclear Security Administration is involved with the Integrated University Program. They provide grants to universities to conduct nuclear security related research.

Beyond this significant investment in nuclear education from the federal government, industry provides funding for nuclear education. Industry provided USD 14 million in scholarships, fellowships, equipment, loaned professors, curriculum development support, internships and equipment to the universities and community colleges in 2010 (NEI, 2012).

## Nuclear education activities

Both private and public colleges and universities provide nuclear education opportunities in the United States. Depending on the location, students can focus their studies into several disciplines that are tied to nuclear science and technology.

The education programmes that are most often focused on are the 25 ABET accredited nuclear engineering and technology programmes (ABET, 2012). These programmes develop students into nuclear engineers and technicians. These programmes are supplemented with schools that focus on health physics programmes that ensure the environment, the population and the workers are kept safe from radiation. Some of the nuclear engineering universities embed heath physics curricula into their programmes, but there are an additional seven universities with health physics programmes in the United States (ABET, 2012).

The ageing workforce has led industry to engage the trade school and community college system in the past four years to develop nuclear energy technology programmes. This partnership has led to the development of 38 trade schools and community colleges working within a network named the Nuclear Uniform Curriculum Program (NUCP) (NEI, 2011). The NUCP prepares graduates for careers in operations, maintenance and radiation protection.

Beyond the energy sector, there are 19 universities with nuclear medicine programmes and close to 100 trade schools and community colleges with radiologist assistant degree programmes that are of significant importance to the nuclear education infrastructure (Education Portal, 2011). These programmes are complimentary to the health physics and radiation protection technician programmes offered in the country. Graduates from these programmes may eventually work outside of nuclear medicine in a laboratory, vendor or utility setting focused on nuclear energy.

One reason the education infrastructure in the United States has been successful is because of the development of networks that support these programmes. The Nuclear Engineering Department Head Organization (NEDHO) is a network of professors that help ensure that nuclear and radiological engineering academic programmes had a forum to discuss, co-ordinate and collaborate on issues facing them (NEDHO, 2012). The Nuclear Uniform Curriculum Program has established a Center of Excellence infrastructure that provides curriculum and graduate placement support to the trade schools and community colleges (NEI, 2011).

Other networks help with research within the university infrastructure. The Oak Ridge Institute of Science and Education provides opportunities for universities to work with the national laboratories on research (ORISE, 2010). They also perform regular enrolment and job placement surveys of nuclear engineering and health physics graduates. The National Organization of Test, Research and Training Reactors (TRTR) focuses on improving US technological competitiveness through education and fundamental and applied research (TRTR, 2012).

Organisations like the American Nuclear Society (ANS) and the Nuclear Energy Institute (NEI) provide support for a wide variety of education and training topics. ANS facilitates a bi-annual conference on Nuclear Training and Education (CONTE) as well as a wide variety of workshops and technical sessions at their annual meetings and several topical meetings such as the biannual Conference on Nuclear Training and Education. NEI facilitates the Nuclear Uniform Curriculum Program which brings together the instructors from the trade schools and community colleges.

## Training activities

A healthy nuclear workforce needs both education and training. Training encompasses the specific information an individual needs to perform a job. Once an individual has graduated from an appropriate education programme and finds an appropriate job matching his/her newly acquired skills, the employee is further trained to conduct the specific tasks he/she is responsible for under the policies and procedures of that organisation. Initial training can be as short as a few days to as extensive as a few years depending on the position and the requirements to become qualified to independently work. Most organisations then provide additional continuing training to employees to keep their skills and knowledge up to date.

In the United States, many skilled tradesmen receive their training through apprenticeship programmes offered by organised labour unions. Journeymen in key trades have their skills recognised through the Nuclear Mechanics Apprenticeship Program (NMAP) (Heyer, 2011). Apprenticeships are multi-year programmes that pay the students to do work alongside fully qualified mechanics until they have gained enough experience to becoming fully qualified themselves. The NMAP helps ensure that apprentices of the seven participating labour organisations receive a uniformly high skill level and a good familiarity with the unique challenges of nuclear power facilities.

The government agencies all have their own initial and continuing training programmes. Following are two examples of specialised nuclear training facilities the US government utilises to develop their employees: the NRC has a specialised Technical Training Center in Chattanooga, Tenn., that includes multiple plant simulators (similar to flight simulators used by pilots) used to train plant inspectors (US NRC, 2012). This allows the inspectors to gain the operational knowledge they need before being an inspector at a nuclear power plant. The DOE has a National Training Center that focuses on nuclear security topics (DOE, 2012b). DOE employees and contractors attend training at the National Training Center to continue their development in safety, security and safeguards related information.

US National Laboratories have been enhancing the quality of the workforce training at each individual laboratory. Proactive measures include: implementing summer school programmes in nuclear-related areas for graduate and undergraduate students; internship programmes; offering nuclear-related degrees for existing employees; entering into long-term partnerships with domestic and foreign universities; supporting selective research fellowships; creating research alliances with universities for grant applications and establishing university research award programmes which are administered by the laboratory to support ongoing mission activities (NEA, 2004).

The US Navy and their contractors hire engineers and scientists to work in their propulsion laboratories, training centers and their Naval Reactors Headquarters. The US Navy also recruits large number of enlisted sailors to work aboard the fleet. All officers and sailors who serve on either a nuclear propelled submarine or aircraft carrier are sent through the US Navy's Nuclear Propulsion School. This training prepares the crew to maintain the nuclear systems of their ship in addition to their normal military duties.

The nuclear energy industry conducts training two different ways. First, each utility conducts its own initial and continuing training of their staff. They conduct this training in accordance with industry guidance and regulatory requirements. The industry then works through the INPO to continuously improve the training regimen.

Each utility maintains 13 accredited and many other non-regulated training programmes. Accredited training includes programmes that cover the engineering, maintenance and operations departments. Training at the utilities can be classroom, laboratory or simulation based. Each site maintains a plant reference simulator which is where a major portion of operator training takes place. These simulators allow the staff to practice evolutions and emergency drills without interfering with normal operations.

The National Academy for Nuclear Training, which operates under the auspices of INPO, embodies the US energy industry's commitment to high quality training and professionalism. In the 1980s as a part of the Industry's Systematic Approach to Training, started after the Three Mile Island accident in 1979, the US nuclear industry developed a Job Task Analysis (JTAs). Its compilation involved both top-down and bottom up approaches and allowed the creation of a "Rubric". The National Academy of Nuclear Training run by INPO maintains these documents and the training guidelines based on the JTAs.

The Academy integrates the training related efforts of nuclear utilities, the Institute's training activities and accreditation. The independent National Nuclear Accrediting Board is responsible for operator and various technical training programmes at every operating plant in the United States. This accreditation carries the weight of NRC regulation and maintaining training accreditation through the National Academy for Nuclear Training is a requirement of the operating license of every utility. In addition, the National Academy for Nuclear Training conducts a variety of training courses and seminars for nuclear plant personnel each year to foster increased professionalism and performance.

## International co-operation

With such a large nuclear education and training infrastructure, many other countries look for opportunities for their citizens to participate in US programmes. Opportunities are available, but since the events of 11 September 2001, additional restrictions have been placed on student visas and access to nuclear facilities by foreign nationals. These include new mandates regarding export controls and the hiring practices of national laboratories.

The US government supports international collaboration in almost all nuclear-related technologies. The openness of information produced by each international project is governed by the international agreement and the export control rules of each participating country (NEA, 2004). The United States are the largest supporter of the IAEA and foster, through IAEA activities, infrastructure support programmes for countries who are interested in building new nuclear power plants.

Since 2001, the domestic scene has stabilised and improved and effort has continued to support collaboration internationally. One of the international efforts of DOE has been the International Student Exchange Program (ISEP) where graduate students from France, Germany and Japan study at a national laboratory in the United States (usually Argonne) while US students study abroad in these three countries. This programme has operated continuously for decades. Other programmes emphasising training in nuclear security and safeguards are offered to domestic and international participants by the State Department and national laboratories.

## References

ABET (2012), *Accredited Program Search*, Retrieved 2 February 2012, from ABET: http://main.abet.org/aps/Accreditedprogramsearch.aspx.

ASME (2011), *Nuclear Stamp Holders*, American Society of Mechanical Engineers, September 2011, Retrieved on 2 February 2012 from: https://caconnect.asme.org/CertificateHolderSearch.aspx.

DOE (2011), *National Training Center*, Department of Energy, Washington, D.C., United States, Retrieved 2 February 2012, available on http://ntc.doe.gov/.

DOE (2012a), Peter Lyons, presentation at NEI Nuclear Research Summit, Washington, D.C. February 2012.

DOE (2012b), *Department of Energy National Training Center*, Department of Energy, Washington, D.C., United States, Retrieved 2 February 2012, available on http://ntc.doe.gov/vid/nelt/.

Education Portal (2011), *Nuclear Medicine Schools*, 6 November, Retrieved from Education Portal: http://education-portal.com/nuclear_medicine_schools.html.

Heyer, J. (2011), NMAP process, Presentation at the Nuclear Talent Taskforce Meeting, Washington, D.C.

IUP (2009), US Public Law 111-8 Division C, Omnibus Appropriation Act, Integrated University Program.

NEA (2000), *Nuclear Education and Training: Cause for Concern?*, OECD, Paris, France.

NEA (2004), *Nuclear Competence Building*, OECD, Paris, France.

NEDHO (2012), *About Us*, Nuclear Engingeering Department Head Organization, Retrieved 6 February 2012, available on http://www-ners.engin.umich.edu/NEDHO/index.html.

NEI (2010), *2010 Nuclear Workforce Report*, Nuclear Energy Institute, Washington, D.C., United States.

NEI (2011), *2011 Nuclear Workforce Report*, Nuclear Energy Institute, Washington, D.C., United States.

NEI (2012), *How Do I Obtain a Career in the Nuclear Industry*, Nuclear Energy Institute, Washington, D.C., United States, Retrieved 5 February 2012, available on www.nei.org/resourcesandstats/documentlibrary/newplants/factsheet/careerhelp/.

ORISE (2011), *Nuclear Engineering Enrollments and Degrees Survey, 2010 Data*, June, Oak Ridge Institute for Science and Education, Knoxville, Tennessee, United States.

SNM (2012), *What Is Nuclear Medicine*, Society of Nuclear Medicine, Retrieved 6 February 2012, available on http://interactive.snm.org/docs/whatisnucmed.pdf

TRTR (2012), *National Organization of Test Research and Training Reactors*, Retrieved 6 February 2012, available on www.trtr.org/ .

US NRC (2011), *US NRC Information Digest 2011-2012*, NUREG 1350 V23, NRC, August 2011, Washington, D.C.

US NRC (2012), *Technical Training Center*, US Nuclear Regulatory Commission, Retrieved 6 February 2012, available on www.nrc.gov/about-nrc/locations/training.html.

*Appendix 3*

# Survey on the use of nuclear research facilities for education and training

To assess the present use of the nuclear research infrastructure for E&T purposes, a survey has been undertaken within the frame of this study, as to date no comprehensive quantitative information has been reported yet on the topic for NEA member countries. This investigation builds on a recent activity developed within the EU Sustainable Nuclear Energy Technology Platform (SNE-TP, 2010).

In order to obtain reliable factual data, owners or operators of facilities were directly requested information by means of the questionnaire reproduced at the end of this appendix. The questionnaire was aimed at gathering numerical data on the access registered historically in research reactors or critical assemblies as well as to thermal-hydraulic test facilities. Information was requested in terms of hours of lab sessions per year, number of students per year, average number of theses per year, over the last five years. Two educational levels were considered: the doctoral and the master levels, as well as general civilian training. Furthermore, the potential capacity of facilities was investigated by asking the respondents to give an estimate of the maximum number of students that may be accommodated in one year in the facility; comments and suggestions for its better use were also sought.

It should be highlighted, however, that no explicit distinction between PhDs researching in nuclear engineering topics and those working on other subjects, such as on solid state or material science was possible though the questionnaire. Thus, the numbers obtained for PhDs theses may not accurately reflect the situation related to nuclear engineering E&T.

Information related to some 230 institutions was obtained, from 21 NEA member countries (including those EU countries covered in SNE-TP, 2010). It should be noted that no numerical data could be obtained on research facilities in the United States. However, an illustration of the situation with regard to E&T uses of US research facilities was provided by Gil Brown, based on firsthand knowledge and experience (Brown, 2011); this is reported in Section 2.3.

Table A3.1 summarises some of the detailed quantitative data gathered through the investigation, the main outcomes of which are further analysed in Section 2.3. It should be noted that no attempt has been made to assess availability and needs for the broader use of research infrastructure for nuclear science and technology, or to provide a comprehensive assessment on the status of ageing of research facilities.

It is the intent of the expert group to incorporate the newly gathered information on E&T uses of facilities in the Research and Test Facility Database (RTFDB). [1]

1. www.oecd-nea.org/rtfdb/.

**Table A3.1: Data on the use of research reactors and critical assemblies for nuclear education**

| Country | Name | PhD | BSc and MSc | | | | | |
|---|---|---|---|---|---|---|---|---|
| | | # PhD (5 years) | Y/N | Lab. sess. Lab. hrs./y. | # students per year | % foreign | Max. # students/y | MSc theses (5 years) |
| **ASIA** | | | | | | | | |
| Japan | JOYO | 3 | Y | 3 = 300 h | 15 | 15 | 30 | 75 |
| | MONJU | 0 | Y | 2 to 4 = 30 to 40 h | 3 to 5 | 0 | 6 to 7 | 12 |
| | HTTR | Currently not used for education purposes. The HTTR could be used for training of the HTGR operator or education of students in the field of basic reactor physic or reactor dynamics. For such use(s) reactor licensing needs should be amended as necessary. | | | | | | |
| | JRR-3 | Y – no records | N | – | – | – | – | – |
| | JRR-4 | N/A | Y | 3 = 64 h | 16 | 0 | 32 | 48 |
| | KURRI-KUCA | 20 | Y | 200 h | 150 | 20 | 200 | 20 |
| | KURRI-KUR | 18 | Y | 35 h | 20 to 25 | 5 to 10 | 50 | 25 |
| | NSRR | Currently not used for E&T – but it could be made available for such use. | | | | | | |
| | FCA | Currently not used for E&T and could not be made available for such purposes. | | | | | | |
| | STACY, TRACY | Currently not used for E&T purposes. These facilities could be used for E&T of students majoring in reactor physics or criticality safety. For such use(s) adjustments of the research and education plan would be required, as well as support for experiment preparation. | | | | | | |
| | TCA | Currently not used for E&T purposes. This facility has been used more than 40 years, and replacements of main components are necessary for long-term utilisation. | | | | | | |
| | Univ. Tokyo YAYOI | 5 to 10 | Y | 5 = 150 h | 15 to 20 | 10 | N/A (shutdown) | 25 to 30 |
| Korea | HANARO | 0 | Y | 6 = 240 h | 300 | 0 | (300) | 0 |
| **OCEANIA** | | | | | | | | |
| Australia | OPAL | 96[2] | Currently used for E&T. Designed to fulfill commercial and research activities it could be used for broader education in nuclear engineering. Funding would be needed to provide external training, which would need to be scheduled in such a way that it would fit with the overall utilisation requirements. | | | | | |
| **EUROPE 27+** | | | | | | | | |
| Austria | TRIGA II | 25 | Y | 8 = 192 h | 60 | 15 | 60 | 50 |
| Belgium | BR1 | 13 | Y | 10 = 40 to 80 h | 40 to 60 | 10 | 240 | 19 |
| | BR2 | | N | – | – | – | – | |
| | VENUS/G | | N | – | – | – | – | |
| Bulgaria | IRT-2000 | 0 | N | – | – | – | – | - |
| Czech Republic | LR-0, LVR-15 | 3 | N | – | – | – | – | 5 |
| | VR-1 | 17 | y | 145 = 435 h | 260 | ? | 700 | 42 |
| Finland | FiR-1 | 3 | Y | 5 = 100 h | 80 | 45 | 150 | 4 |
| France[3] | OSIRIS | 180 | Y | 0 | 0 | 0 | 0 | 2 |
| | ISIS | | Y | 100 = 300 h | 140 | 10 | 200 sessions of 10 students | 0 |
| | MINERVE | | Y | 15 = 45 h | 46 | ? | 100 | 0 |
| | AZUR | | Y | 40 = 120 h | Military training | | | |

2. In the last 12 months for neutron scattering research. Prior to this, only limited neutron facilities were available for PhD students.

3. Other critical mockups run by CEA such as EOLE and MASURCA in Cadarache, SILENE, CALIBAN, PROSPERO and the B Apparatus in Valduc are used for research on criticality, core physics and fuel but no significant use for education purposes is reported.

| Country | Name | PhD | BSc and MSc | | | | | |
|---|---|---|---|---|---|---|---|---|
| | | # PhD (5 years) | Y/N | Lab. sess. Lab. hrs./y. | # students per year | % foreign | Max. # students/y | MSc theses (5 years) |
| Germany | AKR-2 | 5 | Y | 40 = 120 h | 720 | 10 | 800 | 3 |
| | SUR FURT | 0 | Y | 60 h | 50 | – | 100 | 0 |
| | SUR STUT | 0 | Y | 50 = 60 h | 200 | 10 | 300 | 1 |
| | SUR ULM | 0 | Y | 100 = 200 h | 220 | 22 | 300 | 1 |
| | FRM-II | Not used for teaching at master level. However a few PhD theses are related to the core and fuel design changes required by the conversion to LEU. | | | | | | |
| | FRMZ | No data available – used for education in neutron activation analyses, radiation protection measurements and practical training in reactor physics and reactor operation. | | | | | | |
| | BER II | Not used for nuclear technology E&T. | | | | | | |
| Greece | GRR-1 | 2 | Y | 1 = 5 h | 8 | 0 | – | 15 |
| | GR-B | 3 | Y | 12 = 36 h | 220 | 0 | 220 | 5 |
| Hungary | Training R | 5 | Y | 150 = 600 h | 180 | 20 | 300 | 34 |
| | BRR | 15 | Y | 0 | 0 | 0 | 10 | 5 |
| | TR SS MTR | 0 | Y | 16 h | 40 | NR | NR | 0 |
| Italy | AGN 201 C | 0 | Y | 2 = 20 h | 5 | 0 | 10 | 2 |
| | LENA TRIG | 7 | Y | 5 = 20 h | 25 | 5 | 75 | 6 |
| | RSV TAPIRO | 3 | Y | 4 = 32 h | 25 | 0 | 30 | 3 |
| | TRIGA RC1 | 3 | Y | 13 = 80 h | 45 | 0 | 75 | 8 |
| | NEPTUNE Rolls-Royce Marine Power Operations | Currently not used for education purposes – but only for internal train and to a lesser extent other specialist training in naval programmes. | | | | | | |
| Netherlands | HFR | 1 | Y | ? | | | | |
| | LFR | 1 | Y | 48 h | 32 | ? | 32 | 0 |
| | HOR | 50 | Y | ? | 20 | ? | 40 | 20 |
| | DELPHI | ? | Y | 80 h | 20 | ? | 40 | 0 |
| Norway | Halden HBWR | 0 | N | – | – | – | – | |
| | JEEP-2 | 0 | N | – | – | – | – | |
| Portugal | RPI | 12 | Y | 10 h to 30 h | 12 | 26 | 22 | 1 |
| Romania | TR ACPR | 0 | N | – | – | – | – | |
| | TR SS MTR | 0 | Y | 16 h | 40 | NR | NR | 0 |
| Slovenia | TRIGA II | 5 | Y | 3 to 5 = 100 h | 30 | 5 to 10 | 100 | 150 |
| Switzerland | PROTEUS | 4 | N | – | – | – | – | – |
| | CROCUS | 0 | Y | 70 = 150 h | 120 | 10 | 150 | 2 |
| | AGN-211-P | 0 | Y | 90 h | 80 | 0 | 80 | 0 |

## References

Brown, G. (2011), Private communication from Gilbert Brown, University of Massachusetts, United States.

SNE-TP (2010), *Current and Future Uses of Nuclear Infrastructure in Europe*, SNE-TP – Working Group ETKM – Subgroup 4.

# Questionnaire

## 1. Background

It has been identified on many occasions that human resources is one of the most important elements for nuclear energy deployment, with sufficient and assured expertise needed not only for those countries developing new/additional nuclear power, but even for some non-nuclear-power countries and those phasing out nuclear power – to operate and then decommission existing plants and manage radioactive waste. In this context maintaining research activities for both current and future nuclear power utilisation, to be used for the successful transfer of knowledge and "know-how" to the next generation appears key.

The present survey on the uses of nuclear research infrastructure for education and training purposes will form part of a study initiated under the auspices of the Committee for Technical and Economic Studies on Nuclear Energy Development and Fuel Cycle (NDC) of the Nuclear Energy Agency (NEA) of the OECD.

## Information on the use of research facilities for educational programmes

**To be completed by research institutions operating (please tick):**

- Research reactor ☐
- Thermal-hydraulics/severe accident facilities ☐
- Simulator ☐
- Sub-critical assembly ☐

**Completed by:**

Name: Dr. / Mr. / Mrs. / Ms. / Miss / ____________________

Organisation: ____________________

Address: ____________________

____________________

Tel.: ____________________

Fax: ____________________

e-mail: ____________________

| Facility: |
|---|

Q1.1 Vintage of the facilities – Please provide the data below:

- Date of commissioning ____________
- Anticipated or likely shutdown time ____________

Q1.2 Is the research facility used for education or training purposes? (please select)

- Education (please answer questions Q1.3 to Q1.5) ☐
- Training (please answer questions Q1.6 and Q1.7) ☐
- Neither of the above (please answer question Q1.8) ☐

Q1.3 Is the facility used for doctoral research? Y / N

If "Yes", how many PhD students did make use of this facility during the last 5 years?

Q1.4 Is the facility used at bachelor or master level? Y / N

If "Yes", please answer the following questions:

- How many lab sessions are organised per year? Total number of hours of use of the facilities per year?
- How many students benefit from one or several of these lab sessions per year?
- Among these students what is your estimate of the current percentage of foreign students?
- Are they benefiting from a mobility grant?
- If the number of students were to increase, how many students could be accommodated in total in these lab sessions, possibly after increasing the numbers of identical lab sessions?
- How many bachelor/master theses did make use of the facility during the last five years?

Q1.5 Include any suggestion for a better use of the existing facilities that you operate or express the needs for new infrastructures

Q1.6 If the facility is used for training:

- Is it used for internal training only or is it available for others?
- How many people have used the facility per year (on average during the last 5 years)?

Q1.7 Include any suggestion for a better use of the existing facilities that you operate or express the needs for new infrastructures

Q1.8 If your facility is not used for education/training:

- Could it be made available for such purposes?
- If so, at what level (e.g. student trainers that could be accommodated)?
- What would be required for such use(s)?

## *Appendix 4*
# Development of the job taxonomy

A job taxonomy is an in-depth skills classification system which allows the mapping and characterisation of discrete job profiles according to the specific tasks, the responsibilities and activities the role entails, the competencies needed to fulfil them, as well as the associated entry level qualification, training and experience requirements.

This appendix provides some details of the process of development of a framework job taxonomy, which draws on elements of individual national systems of this kind. Several countries have contributed relevant information, gathered, for consistency, by means of common templates issued to all contributing organisations.

The framework taxonomy developed in this study adopts a hierarchical approach, categorising job roles first by sector and secondly by function as described in Figure A4.1.

Sectors are defined by the taxonomy according to the objective for which the workforce is employed, for example, in the nuclear power plant taxonomy, new build, operation, decommissioning and regulation.

Functions are defined by the taxonomy according to the phases or segregated activities within which specific job roles are deployed; for instance maintenance, waste management, safety and environment, operation and control.

*Sectors and functions*

**Figure A4.1: An illustrative taxonomy – sectors and functions**

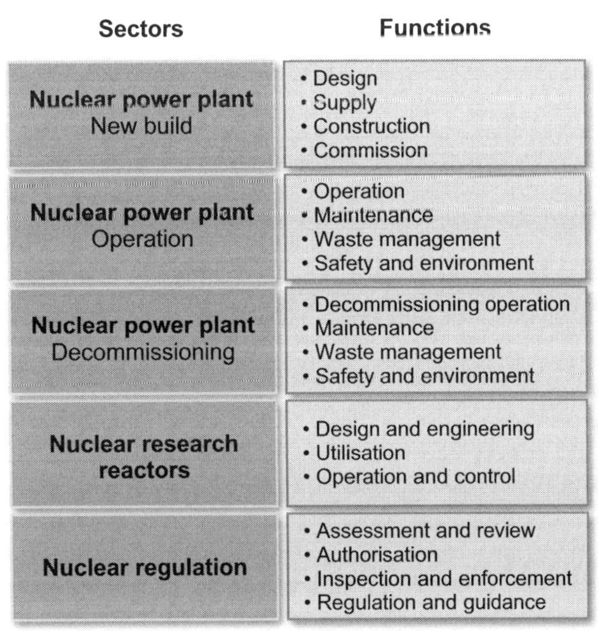

Within each function of each sector, job roles are specified with key competencies at the various occupational levels.

Some job roles that typify each sector and function have been selected for illustration and are listed in Tables A4.1 to A4.4.

Further, a subset of 30 job roles has been distilled for in-depth characterisation. Tables A4.5 to A4.8 list specifications across sectors and functions of the framework taxonomy. The job roles selected for detailed characterisation in each case are deemed as representative and important to the sectors and functions. These are not comprehensive or fully developed and are provided as information advice and guidance on nuclear workforce development.

In order to explain the detailed contents of the tables (A4.5 to A4.8) characterising the job specifications, and to describe the process followed for their derivation, the role of reactor operator for NPP-O (as in Table A4.6) is discussed herein as an illustrative example.

*Reactor operator – An illustrated example*

Six "frames" are used to capture the job specification, namely a frame describing each of the following:

1. header;
2. job title;
3. entry level qualification;
4. job descriptor;
5. competencies;
6. CPD and training.

The title frame outlines the sector, function, occupational level and degree of nuclearisation required for the role [from (*) meaning low nuclearisation to (***) meaning high nuclearisation]. For a reactor operator the title frame thus records NPP-O as the sector, operations as the function, professional as the occupational level, and a high degree of nuclearisation denoted by three asterisks (***).

The frames for the job title and entry level qualification record succinctly the relevant title and qualification together with commonly used alternatives; in this case unit desk operator is an alternative job title, and the qualification is recorded as degree level, although in some cases this can be replaced by stringent nuclear training programmes and substantial experience. This high level of experience means that reactor operators may, in some countries, start out as equipment operators or auxiliary operators supporting maintenance and operation. This allows the trainee to gain experience in NPP operation. With suitable on-the-job training and experience, the trainee may ultimately become licensed as a reactor operator and may become highly qualified in this role.

The job descriptor contains a brief summary of the responsibility and activity. Thus, in the case of the reactor operator, the person is responsible for the manipulation of plant controls from the control room, including monitoring of plant performance, direction of hands-on operations of equipment and performing licensed activities during normal conditions, start-up, shutdown, power changes, emergency and accident conditions, and special configurations. For conciseness and due to variations related to NPP technology, much detail has been omitted as to the precise operations. Some detail is provided in this case to assist the reader.

The reactor operator controls and monitors reactor operations, including power generation, in accordance with plant procedures. This utilises complex instrumentation to control the nuclear reaction which is the source of power (or heat) and which, in turn, is the main mechanism by which the reactor operator maintains voltage and regulates electricity generation from the plant. Control over the reactivity of the core makes the role of reactor operator one of great responsibility, including, in the case of a critical nuclear reactor, shutdown of the reactor. The reactor operator also operates a range of conventional equipment (such as boilers, turbines, generators and auxiliary equipment), e.g. to cater for the distribution of power demand across the reactors of a plant.

 NUCLEAR EDUCATION AND TRAINING: FROM CONCERN TO CAPABILITY, ISBN 978-92-64-17637-9, © OECD 2012

Many NPPs will operate under a "baseload" electricity generation setup, typically close to full power for most of the time, barring maintenance and re-fuelling outages. Nevertheless, when power requirements do change, the reactor operator will power reactors up or down as required. This will typically include computerised control not only to monitor and control the reactor core configuration but also load switching between generators, lines, and transformers. The area which houses the instrumentation and control equipment which the reactor operator uses is commonly known as the control room. It is from the control room that the complex network of automated valves, switches and gauges are operated and monitored. In addition to the reactor operator, there is usually a control room supervisor on duty during each shift.

The above description leads to the required set of competencies which give rise to competence for the job. In the table these are tagged, as explained previously as, technical (T), regulatory (R), business (B) or personal (P). Here, the distinction between "competence" and "competency" is relevant for clarity. Both are much used in the world of business (especially human resource and development).

As has been previously explained, T and R are the most nuclearised of the competencies of a nuclear-related job role. Thus, for the job specification of a reactor operator as illustrated in Table A4.6, T or R appear as tags to all but one of the competencies. The following competency statements for a reactor operator are used here to illustrate that competency may be linked to one or more than one category of competence:

"Advanced fundamental and technical areas, plant design, theory and system interrelationships over which operators have responsibility and control (T)

and,

"Use plant procedures and technical specifications *to implement* appropriate actions under normal, abnormal, and emergency plant conditions (T, R)."

In the former, the competency has been assigned as technical. Here the input, or *competency*, required is the assimilation of knowledge from education, training and experience. These *competencies* can be tested and verified. A combination of prior education (e.g. higher education) and vocational training are commonly used to develop competency in this area.

In many regulated industries the educator or training establishment will also adhere to independent accreditation to quality assure their independence in the application of standards of verification, especially where payment of a fee for education or training may cause conflict of interest in certification of a "customer" or service. This is not an established practice for nuclear for reasons of complexity in T and R.

The competency in either may be tested and certified as before but the interdependence of both the T and the R elevates competency much closer to competence. It is here that experience and CPD combine to create a culture of competence; a culture that may be underpinned by a competence assurance management system.

The final frame of the table captures typical training based on the required minimum standards that can be built upon experience to create a competent reactor operator. Thus, the experienced reactor operator will draw from training and experience in the required competencies (T, R, B and P) to synthesise the competent reactor operator.

## A4.1 Examples of typical nuclear job roles

Table A4.1: Nuclear power plant – new build

| Design | Construction |
|---|---|
| Design leader (P)<br>System designer (P)<br>Reactor core engineer (P)<br>**Design engineer (P)**<br>– **civil**<br>– control & instrumentation<br>– electrical<br>– mechanical<br>**Design technician (T)**<br>– civil<br>– control & instrumentation<br>– electrical<br>– **mechanical**<br>Safety analyst engineer (P)<br>Site layout designer (P)<br>Project manager (P)<br>Planner (T) | **Resident engineer (P)**<br>Civil works engineer (P)<br>Civil construction supervisor (T)<br>Civil construction technician (T)<br>Plant construction engineer (P)<br>Engineering construction supervisor (T)<br>Engineering construction technician (T)<br>**Construction trades (C)**<br>Site quality assurance engineer (P)<br>Quality assurance technician (T)<br>Site inspector (T)<br>Site planner (T) |
| **Supply** | **Commission** |
| **Procurement engineer (P)**<br>Nuclear plant<br>Conventional plant<br>Civil works<br>Quality assurance engineer (P)<br>Inspector procurement (T)<br>Progress control technician (T) | **Commissioning engineer (P)**<br>Nuclear plant testing engineer (P)<br>Conventional plant testing engineer (P)<br>Plant maintenance engineer (P)<br>Plant maintenance fitter mechanical (T)<br>Plant maintenance fitter electrical (T) |

Table A4.2: Nuclear power plant – operation

| Operations (nuclear and non-nuclear) | Waste management |
|---|---|
| Station director (P)<br>**Plant manager (P)**<br>**Operations manager (P)**<br>**Operations technician (T)**<br>Shift charge engineer (P)<br>**Control room supervisor (P)**<br>**Reactor operator/Unit desk operator (P)**<br>Shift plant engineer (P)<br>Fuel handling engineer (P)<br>Operations technician (T)<br>Plant chemistry manager (P)<br>Chemistry technician (T) | Plant waste engineer (P)<br>Waste process technician (T)<br>**Waste operator (C)** |
| **Maintenance** | **Safety and environment** |
| Maintenance manager (P)<br>**Process equipment engineer (P)**<br>Electrical maintenance engineer (P)<br>**Mechanical maintenance engineer (P)**<br>Control & instrumentation maintenance engineer (P)<br>**Process equipment technician (T)**<br>**Mechanical maintenance technician (T)**<br>Electrical maintenance technician (T)<br>Control & instrumentation maintenance technicians (T)<br>**Crafts fitter (C)**<br>IT manager (P) | **Manager health physics (P)**<br>Manager environmental support (P)<br>Radiation protection supervisor (P)<br>Radiation monitor/surveyor (C)<br>Radiation records clerk (C)<br>Security manager (P) |

C: craft occupations; P: professional occupations; T: technician occupations.

Detailed job specifications are given in the following tables for job roles **emboldened**.

## Table A4.3: Nuclear power plant – decommissioning

| Decommissioning operations | Waste management |
|---|---|
| Site manager (P)<br>**Site engineer (P)**<br>**Supervisor/Team leader (T)**<br>**Operator (C)**<br>Planner/Programmer (T)<br>Business (P) | **Operations manager (P)**<br>**Supervisor/Team leader (T)**<br>Support service engineer (P)<br>Operative (C) |
| **Maintenance** | **Safety and environment** |
| Senior engineer (P)<br>Project engineer (P)<br>Team leader (T)<br>Technician (T)<br>**Fitter (C)** | Health physics:<br>– Radiation protection advisor (P)<br>– Health physicist (P)<br>– **Radiation protection supervisor/Team leader (T)**<br>– **Radiation protection health physics surveyor (C)**<br>Safety case:<br>– **Safety case lead author (P)**<br>– Safety case officer (P)<br>– Safety case process owner (P)<br>– Safety case peer reviewer (P)<br>Environment:<br>– Environmental compliance manager (P)<br>– Environmental surveyor (C) |

## Table A4.4: Nuclear research reactor

| Design and engineering | Operation and control |
|---|---|
| Conceptual design and mock-up integration engineer (P)<br>Irradiation engineer (P)<br>Irradiation device design engineer (P) | **Reactor manager (P)**<br>**Reactor operator (T)**<br>**Radiation protection officer (T)**<br>Reactor supervisor **(P)**<br>Shift supervisor (T)<br>Senior reactor operator (T)<br>Reactor operator (T) |
| **Utilisation** | |
| Utilisation manager (P)<br>Utilisation operator and supervisor (P)<br>Target & canning laboratory technician (T)<br>Utilisation scheduler (T)<br>Leader, neutron activation and NAA/DNAA users (P) | |

C: craft occupations; P: professional occupations; T: technician occupations.

Detailed job specifications are given in the following tables for job roles **emboldened**.

## A4.2 Examples of typical nuclear job roles – Specifications[1]

### Table A4.5: Job profiles for nuclear power plant new build

| Civil design engineer | |
|---|---|
| Sector: NPP – New build<br>Function: NPP-NB/Design<br>Occupational level: Professional<br>Nuclearisation: ** | |
| **Job title** | **Entry level qualification** |
| **Civil design engineer** | Degree in engineering, suitable experience, postgraduate qualification desirable. |

**Job descriptor**

The *civil design engineer* is involved in the design, analyses and support to construction for nuclear power plant projects, including civil designs, modifications and upgrades. The individual will be required to support construction of the station and prepare, issue, and execute field-ready design, procurement and construction packages. The types of engineering work may include structural analysis, seismic analysis, detailed design of steel and concrete structures, assessment of existing structures and feasibility studies. The *civil design engineer* prepares and issues design documents, and works closely with the process, mechanical, electrical and other interfacing groups. Duties are carried out under general guidance from the supervisor.

**Competencies** — Technical (T), Regulatory (R), Business (B), Personal (P)

**The *civil design engineer* will be able to:**
- Execute structural and seismic design and analysis work, prepare and issue design documents, and work closely with the process, mechanical, electrical and other interfacing groups. Examples of the kinds of documentation to be produced include design requirements, design guides, design calculations, design reports, design submissions, and technical specifications. (T)
- Assist the supervisor in the preparation of work plans, deliverables, scoping, budgets and schedules. (T)
- Review and comment on the work performed by others. (T)
- Ensure that the work performed meets the quality requirements in accordance with company and business unit QA. (T, B)
- Perform site visits and inspections as and if required in support of design requirements. (T)
- Provide engineering support to field engineering groups. (T)
- Co-ordinate as required from various plant commissioning, operations, and maintenance personnel and client engineering and scientific specialists in interfacing disciplines. (T, P)
- Provide technical guidance to junior civil engineers and/or other technical employees such as technologists, drafting personnel and trades. (T, P)
- Prepare engineering drawing mark-ups, and review engineering drawings pertinent to the design. (T)
- Provide technical support to the clients' safety and licensing organisation and, when and if necessary, participate in discussions with regulators concerning the design in question. (T)
- Participate in formal engineering design and other reviews. (T)
- Control and develop plans and procedures. (T)
- Allocate personnel to activities for the performing organisation. (T, P)
- Monitor implementation of plans and procedures to ensure compliance with project schedules, safety procedures and legislation. (T, R)

**The *civil design engineer* will have:**
- An understanding of the design and analysis of structures gained through the application of civil engineering principles in major construction projects. (R, T)
- Knowledge of nuclear structures, systems and equipment. (T, R)
- Good knowledge of the underlying engineering principles and practices are required. (T, R)
- Working knowledge of national and international design standards and other applicable industry codes and standards in the area of civil/structural design. (R)
- Good technical skills and the ability to seek practical solutions to engineering problems. (R, T)
- Detailed knowledge of one or more of the manufacture, construction and inspection of structural components in a nuclear power plant. (R, T)

**The *civil design engineer* will have:**
- The ability to meet deadlines under pressure. (P)
- A problem solving skills and results-oriented approach and ability. (P)
- Strong planning and organisation skills. (P)
- Demonstrated technical leadership skills including familiarity with a wide range of technical projects. (P, T)
- The ability to network, build relationships, and plan, with an orientation toward service, teamwork and collaboration. (P)
- Excellent oral and written communication skills and a demonstrated ability to effectively interface with staff, project management, customers and regulators as required. (P)
- The ability to communicate complex information. (P)
- The ability to provide learning opportunities for colleagues. (P)
- The ability to manage professional development by setting targets and planning how they will be met. (P)

**The *civil design engineer* may be required to:**
- Understand the theory, principles and practice associated with a variety of business improvement techniques. (B)
- Solve process problems using business improvement techniques. (B)
- Encourage innovation within team. (B)
- Implement quality assurance systems. (B)

| Advised training/CPD | |
|---|---|
| – Licensed to practice in the applicable jurisdiction. (T, R)<br>– NPP fundamentals, NPP design case studies. (T)<br>– Radiation principles. (T)<br>– Internal training in company procedures and practices. (B) | – Risk assessment. (B, T)<br>– Compliance (construction, engineering, nuclear). (R)<br>– Nuclear industry induction, security, context, behaviours. (R)<br>– Safety, health and environmental. (R)<br>– Leadership and management. (P) |

1. The job specifications have been produced on a nominal basis. They are intended to be representative of practice in developing technical and regulatory *safety knowledge and culture*. It is stressed that the competencies and CPD are advisory and do not have regulatory jurisdiction. The examples chosen have been "normalised" for reasons of clarity in terminology and variance in regulatory affairs that naturally occur across an international sample. It is also stressed that for certain roles (not explicitly stated herewith) there is a requirement for a high level of *security* training.

Employment of all roles covered may be subject to security clearance in accordance with national and international regulation.

The title frame outlines the sector, function, occupational level and degree of nuclearisation required for the role [from (*) meaning low nuclearisation to (***) meaning high nuclearisation].

## Mechanical design technician

**Sector:** NPP – New build
**Function:** NPP-NB/Design
**Occupational level:** Technical
**Nuclearisation:** *

| Job title | Entry level qualification |
|---|---|
| **Mechanical design technician** | Vocational qualification in engineering/mechanical technology, and/or suitable experience. |

**Job descriptor**

The *mechanical design technician* undertakes work on mechanical components and systems to ensure compliance with project procedures, quality assurance requirements, schedules, budgets, industry standards and regulations.

**Competencies** — Technical (T), Regulatory (R), Business (B), Personal (P)

**The *mechanical design technician* will be able to:**
- Contribute as a member of a team that provides engineering design, analysis or hands-on work including preparation of design documentation in the area of the mechanical design of the reactor, plant systems and related components. (T)
- Provide technical or hands-on contribution for a variety of equipment including their selection and sizing, support to related development and verification testing, and maintenance, repair, and operation. (T)
- Contribute to documentation including, but not limited to assessment documents, performance analysis, design requirements, design manuals, installation and commissioning documents, registration and equipment technical specifications. (T)
- Assist with recommendations, taking into consideration the feedback from the existing plants as well as client and project requirements. (T)
- Perform general or specific hands-on activities including the operation, maintenance and repair plant equipment or specialised tooling or test equipment and systems. (T)
- Interface with other disciplines as required. (T, P)
- Assist supervision or management with the preparation of detailed planning and budgeting information as required. (T)
- Conduct work in accordance with quality assurance requirements both for safety-related systems, components and structures; and pressure-retaining systems, components and structures in accordance with the applicable codes including the execution of the necessary design verification activities. (T, R)
- Contribute to work plans and resource requirements for the production of deliverables. (T)

**The *mechanical design technician* will have:**
- Familiarity with the design of a range of mechanical components and their design elements relevant to the nuclear industry. (R, T)
- Specific knowledge of some national and international design standards (e.g. ASME) as they may pertain to aspects of the work being undertaken. (R)
- Detailed knowledge of one or more of the manufacture, performance or in-service inspections of nuclear components. (R, T)

**The *mechanical design technician* will have:**
- The ability to understand and consistently meet deadlines under pressure. (P)
- The ability to execute extensive and complex procedures in the performance of specific tasks or activities. (P)
- Effective problem solving skills with a results-oriented approach. (P)
- Skills associated with the performance of a variety of operation, repair or maintenance activities. (P)
- Planning and organisation skills. (P)
- The ability to collaborate effectively in a team environment. (P)
- Good oral and written communication skills and a demonstrated ability to effectively co-operate with staff, project management, and customers if and when required. (P)
- Ability to communicate information in a clear and concise manner and present a compelling case. (P)
- Ability to develop and maintain productive working relationships. (P)
- Open and receptive attitude to change and learning opportunities. (P)
- Ability to manage career development by setting targets and planning how they will be met. (P)

**The *mechanical design technician* may be required to:**
- Understand the theory, principles and practices associated with certain business improvement techniques. (B)
- Support improvements to process problems using business improvement techniques. (B)
- Contribute to and support innovation within the team. (B)
- Comply with quality assurance systems. (B)

**Advised training/CPD** — Technical (T), Regulatory (R), Business (B), Personal (P)

- Membership or certification in a trade organisation. (T, R)
- Trade "passport" schemes as appropriate. (T, R)
- NPP fundamentals. (T)
- Radiation principles. (T)
- Internal training in company procedures and practices with respect to business practices. (B)
- Basic nuclear industry induction, security, contexts, behaviours. (R, T)
- Safety, health and environmental. (R)
- Compliance (construction, engineering, nuclear). (R)
- Supervisor training. (P)
- Leadership and management. (P)

| Procurement engineer | |
|---|---|
| **Sector:** | **NPP – New build** |
| **Function:** | **NPP-NB/Supply** |
| **Occupational level:** | **Professional** |
| **Nuclearisation:** | **** (nuclear plant), * (balance of plant), * (civil works)** |
| **Job title** | **Entry level qualification** |
| **Procurement engineer** | Degree, suitable experience. |

**Job descriptor**

The *procurement engineer* performs procurement functions in accordance with the schedule and technical requirements. In addition, the procurement engineer performs review, verification, approval and acceptance functions as defined within the corporate quality assurance manual programme documents. Extended travel, long hours and a construction environment which will eventually present radiation hazards.

**Competencies** — Technical (T), Regulatory (R), Business (B), Personal (P)

**The *procurement engineer* will be able to:**
- Independently review clients' drawings, technical specifications and prepare technical proposal with completeness, consistency and technical integrity regarding requirements, as well as execute clients' orders with instructions about the general results expected. (T)
- Provide technical guidance and leadership to professionals at lower grade levels and/or other technical employees. (T, P)
- Devise new approaches to problems when preparing technical proposals, cost estimates including preparation of tender documents, request for quotes and selection of successful tenders. (T)
- Develop, plan, schedule, conduct or co-ordinate detailed phases of the procurement engineering work in projects, such as preparation of deliverables including material and documentation, providing packing notes, approved QA release, certificate of conformance/ compliance to logistics for domestic/international projects, updating and maintaining the supplier information database for procurement activities, using information management systems for procurement on engineering, construction, commissioning, and operation work. (T)
- Co-ordinate work of considerable technical and commercial complexity or co-ordinate substantial aspects of large scale projects involving technical review of specifications, review of order (for acceptance), pre-order and post-order project execution including providing training to engineering, drafting, and procurement staff who will use parts of information management systems in their work, and hence providing the information to procurement engineering status during the various project phases. (T, P)
- Define work scope; communicate with clients about engineering requirements, monitor and report progress regarding the administration and maintenance of project procurement engineering identification. (T)

**The *procurement engineer* will have:**
- Familiarity with the design and manufacture of a broad range of mechanical components and systems. (T, R)
- A working knowledge of the applicable national and international standards such as ISO-9000, CSA N285.0, ASME Sections III as well as applicable national regulatory requirements. (R, T)
- Detailed knowledge of one or more of the manufacture, design, construction, performance and operation of nuclear components and systems. (R, T)

**The *procurement engineer* will have:**
- The ability to understand and consistently meet deadlines under pressure. (P)
- The ability to withstand extended travel, long hours and exposure to a construction environment including exposure to radiation hazards that the position involves. (P)
- Effective problem solving skills with a results-oriented approach and ability. (P)
- Strong planning and organisation skills. (P)
- Demonstrated technical leadership skills including familiarity with a wide range of technical projects. (P, T)
- The ability to network, build relationships, and plan, with an orientation toward service, teamwork and collaboration. (P)
- Excellent oral and written communication skills and a demonstrated ability to effectively interface with staff, project management, customers and regulators as required. (P)
- The ability to communicate complex information in a clear and concise manner and present a well structured case. (P)
- The ability to develop and maintain productive working relationships. (P)
- The ability to provide learning opportunities for colleagues. (P)
- The ability to manage professional development by setting targets and planning how they will be met. (P)

**The *procurement engineer* may be required to:**
- Understand the theory, principles and practice associated with a variety of business improvement techniques. (B)
- Solve process problems using business improvement techniques. (B)
- Encourage innovation within team. (B)
- Implement quality assurance systems. (B)

**Advised training/CPD** — Technical (T), Regulatory (R), Business (B), Personal (P)

- Licensed to practice. (T, R)
- NPP fundamentals, NPP manufacture case studies. (T)
- Radiation principles. (T)
- Business improvement (e.g. Six Sigma). (B)
- Risk assessment. (B, T)
- Compliance (construction, engineering, nuclear). (R)
- Basic nuclear industry induction, security, contexts and behaviours. (R, T)
- Safety, health and environment. (R)
- Leadership and management. (P)

| Resident engineer | |
|---|---|
| **Sector:** NPP – New build<br>**Function:** NPP-NB/Construction<br>**Occupational level:** Professional<br>**Nuclearisation:** ** | |
| **Job title** | **Entry level qualification** |
| **Resident engineer** | Degree, suitable experience, postgraduate qualification desirable. |

**Job descriptor**

The *resident engineering* represents the principal link between the design office and the site management and will be responsible to provide technical leadership for areas of expertise and responsibility related to permanently installed reactor components and systems to ensure compliance with project procedures, quality assurance requirements, schedules, budgets, industry standards and regulations.

**Competencies** — Technical (T), Regulatory (R), Business (B), Personal (P)

**The *resident engineering* will be able to:**
- Resolve conflicting technical requirements prior to the onset of installation. (T)
- Anticipate and resolve issues of constructability, communicating with design engineering as necessary. (T)
- Work with design engineering to ensure on-time delivery of information necessary for construction and installation work. (T, P)
- Provide technical support and process the engineering documents supporting installation and construction completion. (T)
- Provide field-engineering input to schedule development. (T)
- Manage the field change process: preparation, evaluation and approval, co-ordination of change implementation, and interfacing with engineering. (T, P)
- Contribute to the preparation of subcontracts and construction work packages in support of field installation activities. (T)
- Develop and implement a process for updating design documents and drawings to their "as-constructed" status. (T)
- Generate site non-conformance reports. (T)
- Provide engineering support for the construction of site facilities. (T)
- In consultation with the site implementation QA manager, ensure delivery of field engineering services in compliance with the project QA manual and site implementation QA plan. (T, R)
- Support personnel safety and ALARA analysis by contributing to reactor component assembly hazard identification and analysis documentation. (T, R)
- Guide and mentor less senior staff as required. (T, P)

**The *resident engineering* will have:**
- An understanding of procedures used for the safe execution of work within an operating nuclear plant. (R)
- Familiarity with the design and installation of a broad range of mechanical components. (R, T)
- A working knowledge of the applicable national and international design standards (e.g. ASME) as well as applicable national regulatory requirements. (R)
- Detailed knowledge of one or more of the manufacture, design, construction, performance and in-service inspection of nuclear components. (R, T)

**The *resident engineering* will have:**
- The ability to understand and consistently meet deadlines under pressure. (P)
- The ability to withstand extended travel, long hours and exposure to a construction environment including exposure to radiation hazards that the position involves. (P)
- Effective problem solving skills with a results-oriented approach and ability. (P)
- Strong planning and organisation skills. (P)
- Demonstrated technical leadership skills including familiarity with a wide range of technical projects. (P, T)
- The ability to network, build relationships, and plan, with a focus on service, teamwork and collaboration. (P)
- Excellent oral and written communication skills and a demonstrated ability to effectively interface with staff, project management, customers and regulators as required. (P)
- The ability to communicate complex information in a concise manner and present a well structured case. (P)
- The ability to develop and maintain productive working relationships. (P)
- The ability to provide learning opportunities for colleagues. (P)
- The ability to manage professional development by setting targets and planning how they will be met. (P)
- The ability to maintain at all times a culture of safety above all. (P, R)

**The *resident engineering* may be required to:**
- Understand the theory, principles and practice associated with a variety of business improvement techniques. (B)
- Solve process problems using business improvement techniques. (B)
- Encourage innovation within team. (B)
- Implement quality assurance systems. (B)

**Advised training/CPD** — Technical (T), Regulatory (R), Business (B), Personal (P)

- Licensed to practice. (T, R)
- NPP fundamentals, NPP new build case studies. (T)
- Radiation principles. (T)
- Business competence and awareness training. (B)
- Compliance (construction, engineering, nuclear). (R)
- Basic nuclear industry induction, security, contexts and behaviours. (R, T)
- Safety, health and environmental. (R)
- Leadership and management. (P)

| Construction trades (process, mechanical, electrical) | |
|---|---|
| **Sector:** | **NPP – New build** |
| **Function:** | **NPP-NB/Construction** |
| **Occupational level:** | **Craft** |
| **Nuclearisation:** | * |
| **Job title** | **Entry level qualification** |
| Trades | Secondary education, vocational programme desirable. |

**Job descriptor**

*Construction trades* perform a variety of skilled and semi-skilled trades at a construction site or development and test laboratory environment, working closely with the process, mechanical, electrical interfacing groups at all levels. The types of work may include the various trade activities such as welding, fitting, wiring, machining, pipe fitting and other labour intensive activities as may be necessary in the construction of equipment or systems. Duties are carried out under the guidance of the supervisor.

**Competencies** — Technical (T), Regulatory (R), Business (B), Personal (P)

**The *trades* will be able to:**
- Perform manual activities associated with the construction at a station site or the development and testing in a laboratory environment. (T)
- Co-ordinate with other trades. (T, P)
- Assist the supervisor in the organisation and execution of the assigned work to complete the entire scope safely, within budget, and on schedule. (T)
- Utilise procedures and drawings as required and complete check lists and other documentation as may be required. (T, R)
- Ensure the work performed meets the quality and other requirements in accordance with procedures and drawings. (T, R)
- Assist in the planning of the work scopes. (T)
- Function as an integral part of the field engineering team. (T, P)
- Obtain inputs as required from various plant commissioning, operations, and maintenance personnel and client engineering and scientific specialists in interfacing disciplines. (T, P)
- Provide feedback as required to draft personnel and engineering on problems or potential improvements. (T, P, B)
- Contribute to plans and procedures as required. (T, R)
- Execute the work to ensure compliance with project schedules, and safety procedures. (T, R)

**The *trades* will have:**
- An understanding of the technical and soft skills required through participation in major construction projects. (R, P)
- Knowledge of the environment and safe practices at a nuclear construction site. (R)
- Good knowledge of the underlying principles and practices as applicable to their particular trade are required. (R, T)
- Working knowledge of site standards and other applicable industry codes in the area of their trade. (R)
- Detailed knowledge of one or more of the trades commonly used at a nuclear power plant. (R, T)

**The *trades* will have:**
- The ability to understand and consistently meet deadlines under pressure (P)
- The commitment to employ safe work practises tailored to and completely suitable for the environment in which the work is being carried out. (R, P)
- Effective problem solving skills with a results-oriented approach and ability. (P)
- Planning and organisation skills. (P)
- The ability to collaborate effectively in a team environment. (P)
- Good oral communication skills and a demonstrated ability to effectively co-operate with staff and management. (P)
- The ability to communicate information in a clear and concise manner. (P)

**In the workplace, the *trades* will:**
- Develop and maintain productive working relationships. (P)
- Be open and receptive to change and learning opportunities. (P, B)
- Manage their career development by setting targets and planning how they will be met. (P)

**The *trades* may be required to:**
- Recommend or support improvements to processes using business improvement techniques. (B)
- Contribute to and support innovation within the team. (B)
- Comply with quality assurance systems. (B)

**Advised training/CPD** — Technical (T), Regulatory (R), Business (B), Personal (P)

- Membership or certification in a trade organisation (T, R)
- Vocational courses in the technical field. (T)
- Trade "passport" schemes as appropriate. (T, R)
- Internal training in company procedures and practices with respect to business practices. (B)
- Compliance (construction, engineering, nuclear). (R)
- Basic nuclear industry induction, contexts, security and behaviours. (R, T)
- Safety, health and environmental (essentials). (R)
- Vocational courses as appropriate. (P)
- Supervisor training (P)

## Commissioning engineer

**Sector:** NPP – New build
**Function:** NPP-NB/Commission
**Occupational level:** Professional
**Nuclearisation:** ** (nuclear plant)

| Job title | Entry level qualification |
| --- | --- |
| **Commissioning engineer** | Degree, suitable experience, postgraduate qualification desirable. |

**Job descriptor**

The *commissioning engineer* performs commissioning functions in accordance with the schedule and technical requirements. In addition, he/she performs review, verification, approval and acceptance functions as defined within the corporate quality assurance manual programme documents.

**Competencies** — Technical (T), Regulatory (R), Business (B), Personal (P)

**The *commissioning engineer* will be able to:**
- Manage technical staff to carry out commissioning of plant structures, systems and components in their designated area of responsibility. (T, P)
- Collaborate with other commissioning groups, operations and project departments as required. (T, P)
- Implement the quality assurance programme for all departmental commissioning activities and prepare and maintain programmatic documents to perform commissioning activities. (T, B)
- Direct the preparation of commissioning documentation such as commissioning specifications and objectives, necessary commissioning procedures, and integrate with the project commissioning schedule. (T)
- Direct preparation and review of proposals for modifications for their systems. (T)
- Ensure production of operational documents and testing procedures to the extent possible during commissioning. (T)
- Certify that the system(s) and components defined in the turnover document packages are complete and all documentation has been provided for commissioning purposes. (T)
- Guide and mentor less senior staff as required. (T, P)

**The *commissioning engineer* will have:**
- An understanding of procedures used for the safe execution of work within an operating nuclear plant. (R)
- Familiarity with the design and operation of a broad range of nuclear and non-nuclear mechanical components and systems. (R, T)
- A working knowledge of the applicable national and international design standards (e.g. ASME) as well as applicable national regulatory requirements. (R)
- Detailed knowledge of one or more of the manufacture, design, construction, performance and operation of nuclear components and systems. (R, T)

**The *commissioning engineer* will have:**
- The ability to understand and consistently meet deadlines under pressure. (P)
- The ability to withstand extended travel, long hours and exposure to a construction environment including exposure to radiation hazards that the position involves. (P)
- Effective problem solving skills with a results-oriented approach and ability. (P)
- Strong planning and organisation skills. (P)
- Demonstrated technical leadership skills including familiarity with a wide range of technical projects. (P, T)
- The ability to network, build relationships, and plan, with an orientation toward service, teamwork and collaboration. (P)
- Excellent oral and written communication skills and a demonstrated ability to effectively interface with staff, project management, customers and regulators as required. (P)
- The ability to communicate complex information in a clear and concise manner and present a well structured case. (P)
- The ability to develop and maintain productive working relationships. (P)
- The ability to provide learning opportunities for colleagues. (P)
- The ability to manage professional development by setting targets and planning how they will be met. (P)
- The ability to maintain at all times a culture of safety above all. (P, R)

**The *commissioning engineer* may be required to:**
- Understand the theory, principles and practice associated with a variety of business improvement techniques. (B)
- Solve process problems using business improvement techniques. (B)
- Encourage innovation within team. (B)
- Implement quality assurance systems. (B)

**Advised training/CPD** — Technical (T), Regulatory (R), Business (B), Personal (P)

- Licensed to practice engineering (T, R )
- NPP fundamentals. (T)
- Radiation principles, protection. (T)
- Business competence. (B)
- Risk assessment. (B, T)
- Compliance (construction, engineering, nuclear). (R)
- Basic nuclear industry induction, contexts, security and behaviours. (R, T)
- Safety, health and environment. (R)
- Leadership and management. (P)

## Table A4.6: Job profiles for nuclear power plant operation

**Plant manager**

**Sector:** NPP – Operation
**Function:** NPP-O/Operations
**Occupational level:** Professional
**Nuclearisation:** ***

| Job title | Entry level qualification |
|---|---|
| Plant manager | Degree in engineering or related science, control room supervisor license/training and suitable experience at managerial level. |

**Job descriptor**

The *plant manager* is responsible for management of overall activities of the operating organisation.

**Competencies** — Technical (T), Regulatory (R), Business (B), Personal (P)

**The *plant manager* will be able to:**
- Schedule and prioritise of work and plan and execution of outages. (B)
- Maintain proper chemistry in liquid systems and compliance with proper radiological requirements. (T)
- Manage costs, work quality and plant availability to meet station performance metrics. (T, B)
- Meet the company's related strategic objectives. (B)
- Comply with the company's quality assurance programme, the station administrative requirements, station procedures and various codes, standards and regulatory guides to which work must be performed. (R, B)
- Ensure all activities are conducted in a safe, cost effective and reliable manner and in full compliance with government regulations, industry best practices and company policies. (R)
- Establish expectations for high levels of performance, monitor performance and reinforce/correct behaviour as required to achieve desired performance. (B)
- Show conservative approach to plant operations. (R, P)
- Exhibit excellent communication skills that foster relationships with all personnel. (P)

**The *plant manager* will understand:**
- How to make conservative decisions, with protection of the health and safety of plant personnel and the public being of highest priority. (P, R)
- Company procedures, programmes and policies and industry guidelines and best practices. (T, R)
- Fundamental and technical areas, plant design, theory and system interrelationships. (R)
- The use of error prevention techniques and human performance tools. (T, B)
- Probabilistic safety assessment concepts and the importance of key equipment to accident mitigation. (T, R)

**The *plant manager* will be responsible for:**
- Providing leadership and strategic focus for all site personnel. (B)
- Communicating expectations, priorities and goals for all site personnel. (B, P)
- Conducting duties required to support the emergency plan. (R)

**Advised training/CPD** — Technical (T), Regulatory (R), Business (B), Personal (P)

- Control room supervisor training programme (fundamentals and technical areas). (T, R)
- Error prevention techniques and human performance tools. (T, B)
- Leadership, interpersonal communication and motivation of personnel. (B)
- Management responsibilities and limits. (B)
- International guidelines and regulations, licensing documentation and technical plant documentation. (T, R)
- Events analysis methodology/operating experience. (T, R)
- NPP emergencies normative and legislation. (R)
- General description of the plant and facilities. (T)
- Station emergency plans. (R)
- Fire protection programme and security programme. (T, R)
- Quality assurance programme. (B)
- Nuclear security, safety and safety culture. (T, R)
- Administrative policies and procedures. (T, B)
- Problem analysis and decision making. (T, B)

| Operations manager | |
|---|---|
| **Sector:** NPP – Operation<br>**Function:** NPP – O/Operations<br>**Occupational level:** Professional<br>**Nuclearisation:** *** | |
| **Job title** | **Entry level qualification** |
| **Operations manager** | Three years degree in engineering or related science together with control room supervisor license and suitable experience or five years degree in engineering or related science together with first year of control room supervisor training programme and suitable experience. |

**Job descriptor**

The *operations manager* is responsible for management of the planning, directing and co-ordinating of the operating activities in accordance with applicable regulations, policies and procedures.

**Competencies** — Technical (T), Regulatory (R), Business (B), Personal (P)

**The *operations manager* will be able to:**

- Perform leadership duties of a manager to ensure safe, efficient and reliable plant operation. (B)
- Ensure all shift operations activities are performed in accordance with requirements of electrical system, local, region and national regulations. (T, R)
- Co-ordinate operations section strategic activities with other sections and operating shifts. (T, B)
- Ensure on-shift personnel are properly qualified. (R)
- Ensure related activities like tagging, technical review of operations procedures, technical specification changes, fire protection testing or radwaste operation are conducted in accordance with plant procedures. (R)
- Control the operation of plant work activities including work package review, input to prioritisation of work, clearance preparation, review and implementation. (T, R)
- Trend and maintain the status of condition reports and corrective actions related to operations. (R, B)
- Show conservative approach to plant operations. (R, P)
- Exhibit excellent communication skills that foster relationships with all personnel. (P)
- Provide leadership and strategic focus for staff. (B)
- Establish expectations for high levels of performance, monitor performance and reinforce/correct behaviour as required to achieve desired performance. (B)

**The *operations manager* will understand:**

- Company procedures, programmes and policies and industry guidelines and best practices. (T, R)
- On-site relationships among different departments (quality assurance, engineering, maintenance, training, radiation protection…). (T, B)
- Fundamental and technical areas, plant design, theory and system interrelationships. (T)
- The use of error prevention techniques and human performance tools. (T, B)
- Probabilistic safety assessment concepts and the importance of key equipment to accident mitigation. (T, R)
- How to make conservative decisions, with protection of the health and safety of plant personnel and the public being of highest priority. (P, R)

**The *operations manager* will be responsible for:**

- The conduct of the operating crews during normal, abnormal and emergency site operations. (R, B)
- Establishing and implementing standardised operation process across the plant. (B)
- The duties assigned to operations personnel. (R)
- The duties assigned to support the emergency plan. (R)
- The procedures related to site operations. (T, R)
- Filling the position of plant manager when plant manager is out of the plant. (R, B)

**Advised training/CPD** — Technical (T), Regulatory (R), Business (B), Personal (P)

- Control room supervisor training programme (fundamentals and technical areas). (T, R)
- Leadership and interpersonal communication. (B)
- Motivation of personnel. (B)
- Problem analysis and decision making. (T, B)
- Administrative policies and procedures. (T, B)
- International guidelines and regulations, licensing documentation and technical plant documentation. (T, R)
- Operating experience. (T, R)
- Management responsibilities and limits. (B)
- Nuclear security, safety and safety culture. (T, R)
- Events analysis methodology. (T)
- Error prevention techniques and human performance tools. (T, B)
- NPP emergencies, normative and legislation. (R)
- Job-related policies and procedures. (T, R, B)
- Radiological health and safety programme. (T, R)
- Station emergency plans and fire protection programme. (R)
- Security and quality assurance programme. (B)

## Operations technician

**Sector:** NPP – Operation
**Function:** NPP – O/Operations
**Occupational level:** Technical
**Nuclearisation:** ***

| Job title | Entry level qualification |
|---|---|
| **Operations technician (also called non-licensed operator)** | High school degree in technical areas. |

**Job descriptor**

The *operations technician* is responsible for operation of the systems and components as directed by a licensed operator or licensed senior operator (control room supervisor).

**Competencies** — Technical (T), Regulatory (R), Business (B), Personal (P)

**The *operations technician* will be able to:**

- Under general directive supervision, perform highly skilled, extremely accurate, complicated operation of selected safety and non-safety related equipment in the power plant. (T, R)
- Perform work of extreme importance in which there is considerable opportunity for making errors having serious consequence to self, others and property. (T)
- Perform work involving hazardous chemicals, potential voltages in excess of 13 800 volts and exposure to health hazards involving radiation requiring special protective equipment; working on or about high pressure and high heat equipment. (T)
- Operate systems locally or from local desks according to plant procedures. (T)
- Monitor the proper functioning of equipment. (T)
- Support fire protection staff when needed. (T, R)
- Perform duties required to support the emergency plan. (R)
- Communicate with main control room before, during and after every duty. (T, P)
- Show conservative approach to plant operations. (R, P)
- Interface with other groups to resolve issues.(P, B)

**The *operations technician* will understand:**

- The scientific principles that apply to the operation of nuclear power plants. (T)
- The importance of confidential, proprietary or safeguarded information. (R)
- The requirements to maintain all the qualifications of a non-licensed operator. (R)
- The use of error prevention techniques and human performance tools. (T, B)
- How to conduct shop briefs and pre-job briefs. (T, B)
- How to make conservative decisions, with protection of the health and safety of plant personnel and the public being of highest priority. (P, R)

**Advised training/CPD** — Technical (T), Regulatory (R), Business (B), Personal (P)

- NPP fundamentals. (T)
- Basic nuclear reactor theory. (T)
- Nuclear technology, plant systems description and plant layout. (T)
- Radiological health and safety programme. (T, R)
- Nuclear security, safety and safety culture. (T, R)
- Job-related policies and procedures. (T, R, B)
- Operating experience. (T, R)
- Industrial safety. (B)
- Error prevention techniques and human performance tools. (T, B)
- Teamwork. (P)
- Conservative decision-making. (T, B)
- Fire protection programme. (R)
- Emergency plan. (R)

## Control room supervisor

**Sector:** NPP – Operation
**Function:** NPP – O/Operations
**Occupational level:** Professional
**Nuclearisation:** ***

| Job title | Entry level qualification |
|---|---|
| **Control room supervisor** | Three years degree in engineering or related science with suitable experience as reactor operator. |

**Job descriptor**

The *control room supervisor* directs operating personnel in all situations that occur to ensure health and safety of the public, as well as protection of plant personnel and equipment. Responsible on a shift basis for safe and efficient plant operation including start-up, shutdown, power changes, emergency and accident conditions, and special configurations as may be required for maintenance or surveillance, etc.

**Competencies** — Technical (T), Regulatory (R), Business (B), Personal (P)

**The *control room supervisor* will be able to:**
- Direct personnel who perform activities on safety related and non-safety related equipment. (T, R)
- Ensure that all shift operation activities associated with power generation are performed in accordance with plant procedures, technical specifications and in accordance with the requirements of the regulator. (T, R)
- Monitor plant conditions and indications closely. (T)
- Control precisely plant evolutions. (T)
- Use procedures effectively in the control of work activities and equipment status and to recognise and mitigate transients and accidents. (T, R)
- Show conservative approach to plant operations. (R, P)
- Interface with other groups to resolve issues. (P, B)
- Perform duties required to support the emergency plan. (R, B)

**The *control room supervisor* will understand:**
- The concepts, philosophy and *control room supervisor* responsibilities with respect to reactivity management and reactor core safety. (T, R)
- Probabilistic safety assessment concepts and the importance of key equipment to accident mitigation. (T, R)
- Fundamental and technical areas, plant design, theory and system interrelationships. (T)
- Transient and accident analyses to determine that procedural actions are effective in maintaining the plant within nuclear safety boundaries during transient and accident conditions. (T, R)
- The use of error prevention techniques and human performance tools. (T, B)
- Supervisory skills to provide effective leadership to a control room shift team to promote teamwork, motivation and positive attitude. (P, B)
- How to make conservative decisions, with protection of the health and safety of plant personnel and the public being of highest priority. (P, R)
- On-site relationships among different departments (quality assurance, engineering, maintenance, training, radiation protection…). (T, B)

**Advised training/CPD** — Technical (T), Regulatory (R), Business (B), Personal (P)

It is assumed that the *control room supervisor* holds unit desk operator license and has passed the associated training programme before starting the following one:
- Supervisory skills. (P, B)
- Error prevention techniques and human performance tools. (T, B)
- Plant procedures and bases. (T)
- Fire protection and operating experience. (T, R)
- Emergency plan. (R)
- Advanced fundamentals in technical areas; system description and reactor operator theory. (T)
- Reactor thermal-hydraulics. (T)
- Technical specifications. (T)
- Radiation protection. (T, R)
- Advanced transient and accident analysis. (T, R)
- Probabilistic safety assessment. (T, R)
- Safety analysis report. (R)
- Simulator training: normal integrated plant operations; emergency procedures; plant transient and emergency response. (T, R)
- Accident management. (R)
- Nuclear security, safety and safety culture. (T, R)

## Reactor operator

**Sector:** NPP – Operation
**Function:** NPP-O/Operations
**Occupational level:** Professional
**Nuclearisation:** ***

| Job title | Entry level qualification |
|---|---|
| **Reactor operator** also known as **unit desk operator** | Degree in engineering or related science and/or stringent nuclear training programmes and substantial experience. |

**Job descriptor**

The *reactor operator* is responsible for manipulation of plant controls, monitoring of plant performance, directing hands-on operations of equipment and performing licensed activities during start-up, shutdown, power changes, emergency and accident conditions, and special configurations. *Reactor operators* principally manipulate plant controls from the control room.

**Competencies** — Technical (T), Regulatory (R), Business (B), Personal (P)

**The *reactor operator* will be able to:**

- Manipulate plant controls in accordance with plant procedures. (T, R)
- Apply theoretical knowledge to practical situations. (T)
- Analyse the operation of equipment in power plant and perform corrective actions for normal and abnormal conditions of equipment according with the plant procedures and the available information. (T, R)
- Use plant procedures and technical specifications to implement appropriate actions under normal, abnormal, and emergency plant conditions. (T, R)
- Place the plant in a safe condition when faced with uncertain or unexpected conditions. (T, R)
- Control and co-ordinate activities of subordinates and others effectively. (R, B)
- Act as an effective member of the control room shift team. (B, R)
- Perform duties required to support the emergency plan. (R, P)
- Show conservative approach to plant operations. (R, P)
- Interface with other groups to resolve issues. (P, B)

**The *reactor operator* will understand:**

- The concepts, philosophy and unit desk operator responsibilities with respect to reactivity management and reactor core safety. (T, R)
- Advanced fundamental and technical areas, plant design, theory and system interrelationships over which operators have responsibility and control. (T)
- On-site relationships among different departments – quality assurance, engineering, maintenance, training, radiation protection. (T, B)
- Administrative procedures and regulatory requirements established for controlling the plant. (T, R)
- Probabilistic safety assessment concepts and the importance of key components to accident mitigation. (T, R)
- Company procedures, programmes and policies and industry guidelines and best practices. (T, R)
- The use of error prevention techniques and human performance tools. (T, B)
- How to conduct shop briefs and pre-job briefs. (T, B)
- How to make conservative decisions, with protection of the health and safety of plant personnel and the public being of highest priority. (P, T)

**Advised training/CPD** — Technical (T), Regulatory (R), Business (B), Personal (P)

- Advanced fundamentals in technical areas, e.g. plant systems description and reactor operator theory. (T)
- Radiological protection. (T)
- Reactor thermal-hydraulics. (T)
  Operating license and technical specifications. (T, R)
- Simulator training: normal integrated plant operations; diagnosis; emergency procedures; plant transient and emergency response. (T, R)
- Probabilistic safety assessment. (T, R)
- Safety analysis reporting. (R)
- Advanced transient and accident analysis. (T, R)
- Mitigating core damage. (T, R)
- Error prevention techniques and human performance tools. (T, B)
- Teamwork. (P)
- Conservative decision-making. (T, B)
- Nuclear security, safety and safety culture. (T, R)
- Operating experience and emergency plan. (T, R)
  Job-related policies and procedures. (T, R, B)

| Process equipment engineer | |
|---|---|
| **Sector:** | **NPP – Operations** |
| **Function:** | **NPP – O/Maintenance** |
| **Occupational level:** | **Professional** |
| **Nuclearisation:** | *** |

| Job title | Entry level qualification |
|---|---|
| **Process equipment engineer** | Four-year (honours) engineering degree with suitable experience postgraduate desirable in suitable areas. |

**Job descriptor**

The *process equipment engineer* is responsible for the maintenance and implementation of repairs or modifications to equipment such as pressure boundary equipment in a nuclear power plant. Examples of such equipment and systems include process valves of all major types, pressure vessels and heat exchangers, rotating machinery, filters and strainers, piping and fittings and miscellaneous equipment.

**Competencies** — Technical (T), Regulatory (R), Business (B), Personal (P)

**The *process equipment engineer* will report to the supervisor and perform duties that may include, but are not limited to the following:**

- Perform critical or major equipment selection and sizing. (T)
- Take a leadership role in preparing equipment-related documentation. This may include preparing equipment assessment documents, performance analyses reports, equipment quotation requests, technical specifications and component spec sheets, bid evaluations and making technical recommendations to purchase. When necessary, certifying the equipment design specifications. (T)
- Perform equipment-related tasks as requested by process system section heads and make recommendations, taking into consideration the feedback from the existing nuclear plants and cost targets. (T)
- Interface with and utilise other discipline groups (such as process design & piping, metallurgy, electrical, C&I, civil) as needed to ensure complete equipment requirements are defined and/or solutions are provided. (T)
- Provide on the job training and mentoring of process equipment staff as required. (T, P)
- Peform the engineering representative duties on major process equipment contracts. This usually involves post award contract engineering, including review and acceptance of supplier drawings and reports, manufacturing inspection and testing procedures, and manufacturing and testing plans, evaluation and acceptance of non-conformances, co-ordination of the review of stress, seismic, vibration and environmental qualification and non-destructive engineering reports, and review and report on the manufacturing progress to anticipate and avert delivery problems. (T, R)
- Lead the engineering interface with suppliers and station staff to resolve equipment problems that may arise during design, manufacturing, testing, installation and operation. (T)
- Take a leadership role in the preparation of concise engineering reports. (T)
- Assist the supervisor in the preparation of work plans and deliverables and ensure adequacy of scopes, budgets and schedules. (T)
- Review and comment on the work performed by others to ensure accuracy, completeness and quality of technical information and design documentation. (T)
- Ensure the work performed meets the quality requirements in accordance with company and business unit QA programmes and manuals. (T, B).
- Perform site visits and inspections as and if required in support of design requirements definition and detailed engineering of design modifications. (T)
- Obtain inputs as required from plant commissioning, and operations engineering and scientific specialists in interfacing disciplines. (T)
- Provide technical guidance to junior engineers and/or other technical employees such as technologists, drafting personnel and trades. (T, P)
- Provide technical support to the clients' safety and licensing organisation and, when and if necessary, participate in discussions with regulators concerning the design in question. (T, R)
- Participate in formal engineering design and other reviews as may be mandated for the designs in question. (T)
- Control and develop plans and procedures. (T, B)
- Allocate personnel to carry out activities within the performing organisation. (T, P)
- Monitor implementation of plans and procedures to ensure compliance with project schedules, safety procedures and legislation. (T, R, B)

**The *process equipment engineer* will have:**

- Practical experience at a nuclear power plant or similar facility or a supplier of similar equipment (required). (T)
- Technical knowledge of process equipment maintenance requirements, functional requirements, design basis and an understanding of process systems in general (beneficial). (R, T)
- Knowledge of materials and metallurgy of materials of construction used in typical nuclear plant process equipment (required). (T, R)
- Knowledge of applicable codes, standards and quality requirements, particularly those specific to this type of equipment is required. (R)
- Practical experience in nuclear plant operation, maintenance, inspection and monitoring (required). (T, R)
- Proficiency with computer systems and tools for the tracking of equipment performance and maintenance data. (T, P)
- An understanding of the safety, security and behavioural expectations of those working on a nuclear site. (R)
- An understanding of the fundamental principles and implications of radiation hazards. (R, T)
- An understanding of the procedures for dealing with radioactive discharges, waste, environmental control and emergency procedures. (R)
- An understanding of the reasons for and application of a variety of safety management systems such as permit to work, standard operating procedures and risk assessment. (R, T)
- An understanding of the implications and relevance of company policy, external legislation and regulation on working practices (including environmental control). (R)
- Personal responsibility for controlling workplace hazards and managing the health and safety of others. (R)
- Personal responsibility to ensure compliance with legal, regulatory, ethical and social requirements. (R)

**In addition, the *process equipment engineer* will have the following skills:**
- The ability to understand and consistently meet deadlines under pressure. (P)
- Effective problem solving skills with a results-oriented approach and ability. (P)
- Strong planning and organisation skills. (P)
- Demonstrated technical leadership skills including familiarity with a wide range of technical projects. (P, T)
- The ability to network, build relationships, and plan, with an orientation toward service, teamwork and collaboration. (P)
- Excellent oral and written communication skills and a demonstrated ability to effectively interface with staff, project management, customers and regulators as required. (P)
- The ability to communicate in a clear and concise manner and present a well structured case. (P)
- The ability to communicate complex information. (P)

**In the workplace, the *process equipment engineer* will:**
- Develop and maintain productive working relationships. (P)
- Provide learning opportunities for colleagues. (P)
- Manage professional development by setting targets and planning how they will be met. (P)

**The *process equipment engineer* may be required to:**
- Understand the theory, principles and practice associated with a variety of business improvement techniques. (B)
- Solve process problems using business improvement techniques. (B)
- Encourage innovation within the team. (B)
- Implement quality assurance systems. (B)

**Advised training/CPD** — Technical (T), Regulatory (R), Business (B), Personal (P)

- Licensed to practice engineering in the applicable jurisdiction. (T, R)
- Radiation protection and regulation. (T, R)
- Nuclear, security, safety, and safety culture. (T, R)
- Safety, health and environmental regulation. (R)
- Internal training in company procedures and practices with respect to business practices. (B)
- Certified compliance with regulatory requirements necessary for the performance of the assigned tasks. (R, T)
- Basic nuclear industry orientation training courses. (R, T)
- Safe work practice training modules. (R)

## Mechanical maintenance engineer

**Sector:** NPP – Operation
**Function:** NPP-O/Maintenance
**Occupational level:** Professional
**Nuclearisation:** ***

| Job title | Entry level qualification |
|---|---|
| **Mechanical maintenance engineer** | Extended degree in engineering or related science, suitable experience. |

**Job descriptor**

The *mechanical maintenance engineer* is responsible for management of the mechanical maintenance programme and maintaining assigned mechanical equipment in a high state of readiness.

**Competencies** — Technical (T), Regulatory (R), Business (B), Personal (P)

**The *mechanical maintenance engineer* will be able to:**

- Manage crews responsible for performing hands-on maintenance following prescribed methods. (T, B)
- Provide leadership and oversee daily maintenance activities to ensure work is performed to appropriate standards using standardised plant practices, policies and procedures. (R, B)
- Prepare and execute refuelling outages in accordance with the business plan. (B)
- Perform emergency response organisation duties as assigned. (R)
- Direct, control and co-ordinate the work activities of company and contractor work force in performing and major mechanical maintenance, including capital modification work. (B)
- Evaluate the maintenance processes and implement standardised changes to optimise maintenance costs, work quality and availability. (B)
- Strategic plan, long range plan for equipment reliability, ensuring adequate staffing, union relations, and setting yearly priorities for the maintenance department. (B)
- Establish high levels of performance, monitoring performance, and reinforcing/correcting behaviour as necessary. (P, B)
- Determine the qualifications for craft advancement and assign number of qualified employees based on maintenance needs. (R, B)
- Show conservative approach to plant operations. (R, P)
- Perform duties required to support the emergency plan. (R, P)
- Conduct condition report generation, investigation and processing. (T, R)
- Assign tasks and manage personnel to ensure due dates and completions standards are met. (B)
- Ensure activities are completed in accordance with standardised plant practices, policies and procedures. (T, R)
- Enforce established site standards and expectations with the workforce by providing in-field oversight, mentoring and coaching for assigned work crews. (P, B)

**The *mechanical maintenance engineer* will understand:**

- Company procedures, programmes and policies and industry guidelines and best practices. (T, R)
- On-site relationships among different departments – quality assurance, engineering, maintenance, training, radiation protection. (T, B)
- Fundamental and technical areas, plant design, theory and system interrelationships. (T)
- The use of error prevention techniques and human performance tools. (T, B)
- How to make conservative decisions, with protection of the health and safety of plant personnel and the public being of highest priority. (P, R)
- How to conduct shop briefs and pre-job briefs. (T, B)

**Advised training/CPD** — Technical (T), Regulatory (R), Business (B), Personal (P)

- Control room supervisor training programme (fundamentals and technical areas). (T, R)
- Leadership. (B)
- Interpersonal communication. (B)
- Management responsibilities and limits. (B)
- Motivation of personnel. (B)
- Problem analysis and decision making. (T, B)
- Administrative policies and procedures. (T, B)
- Station emergency plans. (R)
- Fire protection programme and operating experience. (T, R)
- Nuclear security, safety and safety culture. (T, R)
- International guidelines and regulations, licensing documentation and technical plant documentation. (T, R)
- Advanced fundamentals in mechanical maintenance. (T)
- Error prevention techniques and human performance tools. (T, B)
- General description of the plant and facilities. (T)
- Job-related policies and procedures. (T, R, B)
- Radiological health and safety. (T)
- Security and quality assurance. (B)

| **Process equipment technician** | |
|---|---|
| **Sector:** NPP – Operations<br>**Function:** NPP – O/Maintenance<br>**Occupational level:** Technical<br>**Nuclearisation:** *** | |
| **Job title** | **Entry level qualification** |
| **Process equipment technician** | Three-year engineering technology diploma and/or suitable experience. |

**Job descriptor**

The *process equipment technician* is responsible for the maintenance and implementation of repairs or modifications to equipment such as pressure boundary equipment in a nuclear power plant. Examples of such equipment and systems include process valves of all major types, pressure vessels and heat exchangers, rotating machinery, filters and strainers, piping and fittings and miscellaneous equipment.

**Competencies** — Technical (T), Regulatory (R), Business (B), Personal (P)

**The *process equipment technician* will report to the supervisor and perform duties that may include, but are not limited to the following:**

- Perform critical or major equipment selection and sizing. (T)
- Provide hands-on contribution for a variety of equipment including their testing, maintenance, repair, and operation. This may be plant equipment or tooling for the repair or maintenance of plant equipment. (T)
- Contribute to preparing equipment-related documentation. This may include equipment assessment documents, performance analyses reports, equipment quotation requests, technical specifications and component spec sheets, bid evaluations and making technical recommendations to purchase. When necessary, certifying the equipment design specifications. (T)
- Perform equipment-related tasks as requested by process system section heads and make recommendations, taking into consideration the feedback from the existing nuclear plants and cost targets. (T)
- Interface with and utilise other discipline groups (such as process design & piping, metallurgy, electrical, C&I, civil) as needed to ensure the successful execution of the assigned work. (T)
- Support the engineering interface with suppliers and station staff to resolve equipment problems that may arise during design, manufacturing, testing, installation, operation, repair and maintenance. (T)
- Contribute to the preparation of concise engineering reports. (T)
- Assist with the preparation of work plans and deliverables and ensure adequacy of scopes, budgets and schedules. (T)
- Ensure the work performed meets the quality requirements in accordance with company and business unit QA programmes and manuals. (T, B)
- Perform site visits and inspections as and if required in support of the engineering of design modifications or the performance of inspection, repair or maintenance activities. (T)
- Obtain inputs as required from plant commissioning, and operations engineering and scientific specialists in interfacing disciplines. (T)
- Provide technical guidance to junior technicians and/or other technical employees such as trades. (T, P)
- Contribute to the development of plans and procedures. (T, B)
- Execute extensive and complex procedures in the performance of specific tasks or activities and to ensure compliance with project schedules and safety procedures. (T, R, B)

**The *process equipment technician* will have:**

- Practical experience at a nuclear power plant or similar facility or a supplier of similar equipment (required). (T)
- Technical knowledge of process equipment maintenance requirements, functional requirements, design basis and an understanding of process systems in general (beneficial). (T)
- Knowledge of applicable codes, standards and quality requirements, particularly those specific to this type of equipment (required). (R)
- Practical experience in nuclear plant operation, maintenance, inspection and monitoring (asset). (T, R)
- Proficiency with computer systems and tools for the tracking of equipment performance and maintenance data. (T, P)
- An understanding of the safety, security and behavioural expectations of those working on a nuclear site. (R)
- An understanding at the working level of the implications of radiation hazards. (R, T)
- An understanding of the application of a variety of safety management systems such as permit to work, standard operating procedures and risk assessment. (R, T)
- An understanding of the applications of company policy, external legislation and regulation on working practices (including environmental control). (R)
- Personal responsibility for workplace hazards and the health and safety of others. (R)
- Personal responsibility to ensure compliance with legal, regulatory, ethical and social requirements. (R)

**In addition the *process equipment technician* will have the following skills:**

- The ability to understand and consistently meet deadlines under pressure. (P)
- The ability to execute extensive and complex procedures in the performance of specific tasks or activities. (P)
- Effective problem solving skills with a results-oriented approach and ability. (P)
- Planning and organisation skills. (P)
- The ability to collaborate effectively in a team environment. (P)
- Excellent oral and written communication skills and a demonstrated ability to effectively interface with staff, project management, and customers if and when required. (P)
- The ability to communicate information in a clear and concise manner and present a compelling case. (P)

**In the workplace, the *process equipment technician* will:**

- Develop and maintain productive working relationships. (P)
- Be open and receptive to change and learning opportunities. (P)
- Manage his/her career development by setting targets and planning how they will be met. (P)

**The *process equipment technician* may be required to:**

- Understand the theory, principles and practices associated with certain business improvement techniques. (B)
- Support improvements to process problems using business improvement techniques. (B)
- Contribute to and support innovation within the team. (B)
- Comply with quality assurance systems. (B)

**Advised training/CPD** — Technical (T), Regulatory (R), Business (B), Personal (P)

- Membership and/or certification in a trade organisation authorised to represent technology in the applicable jurisdiction. (T, R)
- Internal training in company procedures and practices with respect to business practices. (B)
- Job-related procedures and practices. (T, R)
- Basic nuclear industry orientation training courses. (R, T)
- Nuclear security, safety and safety culture. (T, R)
- Safety, health and environmental regulation. (R)
- Safe work practice training modules. (R)


NUCLEAR EDUCATION AND TRAINING: FROM CONCERN TO CAPABILITY, ISBN 978-92-64-17637-9, © OECD 2012

| Mechanical maintenance technician | |
|---|---|
| **Sector:** NPP – Operation<br>**Function:** NPP – O/Operations<br>**Occupational level:** Technical<br>**Nuclearisation:** *** | |
| **Job title** | **Entry level qualification** |
| **Mechanical maintenance technician** | Three years degree in engineering or related science. |

**Job descriptor**

The *mechanical maintenance technician* is responsible for the supervision of mechanical maintenance daily activities.

**Competencies** — Technical (T), Regulatory (R), Business (B), Personal (P)

**The *mechanical maintenance technician* will be able to:**

- Supervise and co-ordinate daily mechanical maintenance work on plant equipment and facilities consistent with standardised plant fleet practices, policies and procedures. (T, R)
- Assign tasks and manage personnel to ensure due dates and completions standards are met. (B)
- Supervise and direct craft and contractor personnel in the conduct of maintenance. (B)
- Promptly investigate and settle grievances.(T, P)
- Ensure personnel are properly trained and qualified to perform assigned activities. (R)
- Perform duties required to support the emergency plan. (R)
- Conduct condition report generation, investigation and processing. (T, P)
- Enforce established site standards and expectations with the workforce by providing in-field oversight, mentoring and coaching for assigned work crews. (B)
- Provide on-line and pre-outage work order reviews, walk downs and validation for correctness of scope, parts, clearances and work package preparation. (T, B)
- Interface with other groups to resolve issues. (P, B)
- Schedule implementation during on-line and outage periods. (B)
- Show conservative approach to plant operations. (R, P)
- Perform duties required to support the emergency plan. (R, P)
- Conduct condition report generation, investigation and processing. (T, R)

**The *mechanical maintenance technician* will understand:**

- Company procedures, programmes and policies and industry guidelines and best practices. (T, R)
- The use of error prevention techniques and human performance tools. (T, B)
- How to make conservative decisions, with protection of the health and safety of plant personnel and the public being of highest priority. (P, R)
- Fundamental and technical areas, plant design, theory and system interrelationships. (T)
- How to conduct shop briefs and pre-job briefs. (T, B)
- On-site relationships among different departments (quality assurance, engineering, maintenance, training, radiation protection…). (T, B)

**Advised training/CPD** — Technical (T), Regulatory (R), Business (B), Personal (P)

- NPP fundamentals and industry awareness. (T)
- Basic nuclear reactor theory. (T)
- Nuclear technology, plant systems description and plant layout. (T)
- Advanced fundamentals in mechanical maintenance. (T)
- Radiological health and safety programme. (T, R)
- Job-related policies and procedures. (T, R, B)
- Nuclear security, safety and safety culture. (T, R)
- Safety, health and environmental regulation. (R)
- Industrial safety. (B)
- Error prevention techniques and human performance tools. (T, B)
  Conservative decision-making. (T, B)
- Teamwork. (P)
- Fire protection programme. (R)
- Emergency plan. (R)
- Job-related procedures and practices (T, R. B)

| Crafts fitter | |
|---|---|
| **Sector:** | **NPP – Operation** |
| **Function:** | **NPP – O/Operations** |
| **Occupational level:** | **Craft** |
| **Nuclearisation:** | *** |

| Job title | Entry level qualification |
|---|---|
| **Crafts fitter** | High school degree in technical areas. |

**Job descriptor**

The *crafts fitter* is responsible for performing mechanical maintenance activities.

**Competencies** — Technical (T), Regulatory (R), Business (B), Personal (P)

**The *crafts fitter* will be able to:**

- Check the limits of disclaimers.(T)
- Execute work with the necessary means to ensure minimum radiation exposure and contamination. (T, R)
- Perform work in compliance with the regulations to avoid accidents and human error. (T, R)
- Comply with the procedures applicable in each case, indicating the possible deviations from their supervisors, and suggesting improvements to them. (T, R)
- Execute the tasks in the workshop or field in accordance with existing procedures. (T, R)
- Issue reports to their superiors of deficiencies in the implementation of its work. (T, R)
- Show conservative approach to plant operations. (R, P)
- Interface with other groups to resolve issues. (P, B)
- Perform duties required to support the emergency plan. (R)

**The *crafts fitter* will understand:**

- The scientific principles that apply to the operation of nuclear power plants. (T)
- The use of error prevention techniques and human performance tools. (T, B)
- How to make conservative decisions, with protection of the health and safety of plant personnel and the public being of highest priority. (P, R)

**Advised training/CPD** — Technical (T), Regulatory (R), Business (B), Personal (P)

- NPP fundamentals and industry awareness. (T)
- Nuclear technology, plant systems description and plant layout. (T)
- Basic fundamentals in mechanical maintenance. (T)
- Organisational fundamentals. (T, B)
- Radiological protection. (T, R)
- Nuclear security, safety and safety culture. (T, R)
- Job-related policies and procedures. (T, R, B)
- Industrial safety. (B)
- Error prevention techniques and human performance tools. (T, B)
- Teamwork. (P)
- Conservative decision-making. (T, B)
- Fire protection programme. (R)
- Emergency plan. (R)
- Safety, health and environmental regulation. (R)

| Waste operator | |
|---|---|
| **Sector:** | **NPP – Operation** |
| **Function:** | **NPP-O/Waste management** |
| **Occupational level:** | **Craft** |
| **Nuclearisation:** | *** |
| **Job title** | **Entry level qualification** |
| **Waste operator** | School leaving qualification or vocational qualification in technical area. |

**Job descriptor**

The *waste operator* is responsible for operating panels of the systems involved in collecting and processing of radioactive waste.

**Competencies** — Technical (T), Regulatory (R), Business (B), Personal (P)

**The *waste operator* will be able to:**
- Operate the systems involved in collecting and processing of radioactive waste. (T, R)
- Maintain different parameters of those systems involved in collecting and processing of radwaste in accordance with technical specifications and operating license. (T, R)
- Communicate and co-ordinate with main control room and radiological protection service before a radwaste discharge. (T)
- Monitor the proper functioning of radioactive waste equipment. (T, R)
- Issue reports to superior of deficiencies in the implementation of work. (T, R)
- Perform duties required to support the emergency plan. (R)
- Show conservative approach to plant operations. (R, P)
- Interface with other groups to resolve issues. (P, B)

**The *waste operator* will understand:**
- The use of error prevention techniques and human performance tools. (T, B)
- How to conduct shop briefs and pre-job briefs. (T, B)
- On-site relationships among different departments – quality assurance, engineering, maintenance, training, radiation protection. (T, B)
- The scientific principles that apply to the operation of nuclear power plants. (T)
- How to make conservative decisions, with protection of the health and safety of plant personnel and the public being of highest priority. (P, R)

**Advised training/CPD** — Technical (T), Regulatory (R), Business (B), Personal (P)

- NPP fundamentals and industry awareness. (T)
- Nuclear technology, plant systems description and plant layout. (T)
- Advanced fundamentals in radioactive waste systems. (T)
- Radiological protection. (T, R)
- Organisational fundamentals. (T, B)
- Nuclear security, safety and safety culture. (T, R)
- Job-related policies and procedures. (T, R, B)
- Industrial safety. (B)
- Error prevention techniques and human performance tools. (T, B)
- Teamwork. (P)
- Conservative decision-making. (T, B)
- Fire protection programme. (R)
- Safety, health and environmental regulation. (R)
- Emergency plan. (R)

## Manager, health physics

**Sector:** NPP – Operation
**Function:** NPP-O/Safety
**Occupational level:** Professional
**Nuclearisation:** ***

| Job title | Entry level qualification |
|---|---|
| **Manager, health physics** | Degree in engineering or related science, first year of control room supervisor training programme, suitable experience. |

**Job descriptor**

The *health physics manager* is responsible for management of the radiological protection programme.

**Competencies** — Technical (T), Regulatory (R), Business (B), Personal (P)

**The *manager, health physics* will be able to:**

- Manage all aspects of radiation protection in conformance to regulations and nuclear industry standards. (T, R)
- Plan and control all aspects of radiation protection initiatives. (T, R)
- Direct, control and co-ordinate the activities of the RP section to meet station performance metrics. (T, B)
- Assign tasks and manage personnel to ensure due dates and completions standards are met. (T)
- Ensure activities are completed in accordance with standardised plant practices, policies and procedures. (T, R)
- Ensure satisfactory performance and qualification of assigned personnel; develop assigned personnel for increased responsibility and more demanding projects. (R, B)
- Exhibit excellent communication skills that foster relationships with all personnel. (P)
- Provide regulatory requirements regarding radiation safety. (R)
- Provide support for station operations and maintenance activities. (B)
- Ensure the preparation and adequacy of personnel exposure records, bioassay samples and radiation and contamination surveys to assure plant personnel radiation exposure is kept as low as reasonably achievable (ALARA). (T, R)
- Ensure the timely preparation and maintenance of records and reports concerning radiation and radioactive material as required by national, regional and local agencies. (R)
- Comply with the company's quality assurance programme, administrative requirements, radiological control procedures and various codes, standards and regulatory guides to which radiological activities must be performed. (R)
- Perform duties required to support the emergency plan. (R, P)
- Provide leadership and strategic focus for staff. (P, B)
- Establish high levels of performance, monitor performance and reinforce/correct behaviour as necessary. (B)
- Manage and complete assigned activities to support timely implementation of required site operations. (P, B)
- Interface with other groups to resolve issues. (P, B)
- Show accountable for training qualification and performance of section personnel. (P, B)
- Show conservative approach to plant operations. (R, P)
- Communicate expectations, priorities and goals for staff. (P, B)

**The *manager health physics* will understand:**

- Responsibilities for maintaining open communications and responsive co-ordination with all other station organisations, regulators and site management for effective implementation of the radiation programme. (P, B)
- How to make conservative decisions, with protection of the health and safety of plant personnel and the public being of highest priority. (P, R)
- Fundamental and technical areas, plant design, theory and system interrelationships. (T)
- The use of error prevention techniques and human performance tools. (T, B)
- How to conduct condition report generation, investigation and processing. (T, R)
- Company procedures, programmes and policies and industry guidelines and best practices. (T, R)

**Advised training/CPD** — Technical (T), Regulatory (R), Business (B), Personal (P)

- Radiation protection licence. (T, R)
- Leadership. (B)
- Interpersonal communication. (P, B)
- Management responsibilities and limits. (B)
- Motivation of personnel. (B)
- Problem analysis and decision-making. (T, B)
- Administrative policies and procedures. (T, B)
- Security and quality assurance programme. (B)
- Events analysis methodology. (T)
- Radiological health and safety. (T, R)
- Nuclear security, safety and safety culture. (T, R)
- International guidelines and regulations, licensing documentation and technical plant documentation. (T, R)
- Error prevention techniques and human performance tools. (T, B)
- General description of the plant and facilities. (T)
- Job-related policies and procedures. (T, R, B)
- Station emergency plans. (R)
- Fire protection programme.. (T, R)
- Safety, health and environmental regulation. (R)

### Table A4.7: Job profiles for nuclear power plant decommissioning

| Site engineer | |
|---|---|
| **Sector:** | **NPP – Decommissioning (lead: United Kingdom)** |
| **Function:** | **NPP-D/Decommissioning operations** |
| **Occupational level:** | **Professional** |
| **Nuclearisation:** | *** |
| **Job title** | **Entry level qualification** |
| **Decommissioning site engineer** also known as **decommissioning implementation engineer** | Degree in engineering or physical science or substantial suitable experience. |

**Job descriptor**

The *decommissioning site engineer* allocates personnel to prepare for/carry out decommissioning operations, monitoring implementation of plans and procedures to ensure compliance with project schedules, safety procedures and legislation. The engineer controls and develops plans and procedures, and responds to and resolves problems arising during decommissioning operations.

**Competencies** — Technical (T), Regulatory (R), Business (B), Personal (P)

**The *decommissioning site engineer* will be able to:**
- Control and develop plans and procedures. (T)
- Allocate personnel to prepare for/carry out decommissioning operations. (T, P)
- Respond to and solve decommissioning problems. (T, P)
- Monitor implementation of plans and procedures to ensure compliance with project schedules, safety procedures and legislation. (T, R, B)

**Additionally the *decommissioning site engineer* may be required to:**
- Instigate decommissioning plans. (T)

**The *decommissioning site engineer* will understand:**
- Radioactivity and nuclear science and engineering. (T)
- Methods of decontamination. (T)
- How to fix high activity, mobile contamination. (T)
- The range of manual and remote dismantling techniques, benefits and challenges. (T)

**The *decommissioning site engineer* will understand:**
- The safety, security and behavioural expectations of those working on a nuclear site. (R)
- The fundamental principles of and implications of radiation hazards. (R, T)
- The construction of, and standards used, in a modern standards decommissioning safety case. (R, T)
- The procedures for dealing with radioactive discharges, waste, environmental control and emergency procedures. (R, T)
- The reasons for and application of a variety of safety management systems such as permit to work, standard operating procedures and risk assessment. (R, T)
- The implications and relevance of company policy, external legislation and regulation on working practices (including environmental control). (R)
- Personal responsibility for controlling workplace hazards and managing the health and safety of others. (R)
- Personal responsibility to ensure compliance with legal, regulatory, ethical and social requirements. (R)

**The *decommissioning site engineer* will:**
- Develop and maintain productive working relationships. (P)
- Provide learning opportunities for colleagues. (P)
- Manage professional development by setting targets and planning how they will be met. (P)
- Communicate in a clear and concise manner and present a well structured case. (P)
- Communicate complex information. (P)
- Handover at end of shift. (P)

**The *decommissioning site engineer* may be required to:**
- Understand the theory, principles and practice associated with a variety of business improvement techniques. (B)
- Solve process problems using business improvement techniques. (B)
- Encourage innovation within team. (B)
- Implement quality assurance systems. (B)

**Advised training/CPD** — Technical (T), Regulatory (R), Business (B), Personal (P)

- Nuclear industry awareness, context and behaviours. (T, R)
- Science and engineering of nuclear decommissioning. (T)
- Principles of ionising radiation. (T)
- Radiological protection. (T, R)
- Business improvement. (B)
- Risk assessment and safety management. (B, T)
- Nuclear industry awareness, context, behaviours, regulations. (R)
- Nuclear regulation compliance. (R)
- Safety, health and environmental legislation. (R)
- Leadership and management. (P)
- Quality assurance. (T, R)
- Safety case analysis. (T)
- Nuclear security, safety and safety culture. (T, R)
- Job-related policies and procedures. (T, R, B)

## Decommissioning supervisor

**Sector:** NPP – Decommissioning
**Function:** NPP-D/Decommissioning operations
**Occupational level:** Technical
**Nuclearisation:** ***

| Job title | Entry level qualification |
|---|---|
| **Decommissioning supervisor** also known as **decommissioning team leader** | Vocational qualification (technical area). |

**Job descriptor**

The *decommissioning supervisor* reports to the decommissioning site engineer and is responsible for the safe and efficient management of a team undertaking nuclear decommissioning activities. The supervisor/team leader manages, implements and monitors plant, equipment and personnel within scope of authority and ensures that health and safety legislative requirements are adhered to.

**Competencies** — Technical (T), Regulatory (R), Business (B), Personal (P)

**The *decommissioning supervisor* will be able to:**
- Demonstrate a thorough understanding of nuclear decommissioning practices. (T)
- Take a leading role in contributing to ideas for the control and implementation of work. (T)
- Allocate work effectively and fairly to the decommissioning team and supervise radiation related work activities. (T, R, P)
- Manage a team delivering a decommissioning project, ensuring that key objectives are achieved. (T, P)
- Implement safe access systems in a radiation/contamination controlled environment. (T, R, P).
- Enable learning within team, through demonstration, instruction and coaching. (T, P)

**The *decommissioning supervisor* will understand:**
- Practice involved with the optimisation, packaging and removal of hazardous materials and their transfer to designated storage areas. (T, R)

**The *decommissioning supervisor* will understand:**
- Safety, security and behavioural expectations of those working on a nuclear site. (R)
- Fundamental principles of and implications of radiation hazards. (R, T)
- Procedures for dealing with radioactive discharges, waste, environmental control and emergency. (R)
- Reasons for and application of a variety of safety management systems such as permit to work, standard operating procedures and risk assessment. (R, T)
- Implications and relevance of company policy, external legislation and regulation on working practices (including environmental control). (R)

***The decommissioning supervisor* will have:**
- Good communications, numeracy, IT skills. (P)
- Responsibility for competing tasks and procedures. (P)
- Autonomy and judgement subject to overall direction or guidance. (P)
- Co-operative relationships. (P)
- The ability to plan work with others and review progress against objectives. (P)
- The ability to contribute to improvement of collaborative working. (P)
- The responsibility for supervising or guiding others where appropriate. (P)
- The responsibility for personal development by setting targets and planning how they will be met, reviewing progress towards targets and establishing evidence of achievements. (P)
- The ability to communicate complex information to others. (P)
- Handover at end of shift. (P)

**The *decommissioning supervisor* may be required to:**
- Apply a variety of appropriate business improvement to solve problems and improve efficiency. (B)
- Solve routine decommissioning problems using business improvement techniques. (B, T)
- Understand the theory principles and practice associated with a variety of appropriate business improvement techniques. (B)

**Advised training/CPD** — Technical (T), Regulatory (R), Business (B), Personal (P)

- Science and engineering of nuclear decommissioning. (T)
- Principles of ionising radiation. (T)
- Radiological protection. (T, R)
- Business improvement. (B)
- Risk assessment and management. (B, T)
- Safety management systems. (R)
- Nuclear industry awareness, context, behaviours, regulations. (T, R)
- Nuclear regulation compliance. (R)
- Safety, health and environmental legislation. (R)
- Leadership and management. (B, P)
- Job-related policies and procedures. (T, R, B)

 NUCLEAR EDUCATION AND TRAINING: FROM CONCERN TO CAPABILITY, ISBN 978-92-64-17637-9, © OECD 2012

| Operator | |
|---|---|
| **Sector:** NPP – Decommissioning<br>**Function:** NPP-D/Decommissioning operations<br>**Occupational level:** Craft<br>**Nuclearisation:** *** | |
| **Job title** | **Entry level qualification** |
| **Decommissioning operator** also known as **decommissioning operative** | Secondary education, vocational programme desirable. |

**Job descriptor**

The *decommissioning operator* controls and operates basic decommissioning plant and equipment efficiently and safely. The individual reports and investigates deviations from routine operating conditions and deals with basic process upsets. Capable of minimising and transferring waste and associated decommissioning matters arising.

**Competencies** — Technical (T), Regulatory (R), Business (B), Personal (P)

**The *decommissioning operator* will be able to:**
- Prepare work area for decommissioning activities. (T)
- Assemble, dismantle, operate, maintain, monitor and adjust, equipment. (T)
- Dismantle contaminated plant, structures and equipment. (T)
- Decontaminate radioactive plant and materials. (T)
- Minimise and package radioactive materials. (T)
- Remove and transfer hazardous materials to designated storage locations. (T)

**Additionally, the *decommissioning operator* may be required to:**
- Support and prepare alpha, beta/gamma radiation contamination controlled work areas. (T)
- Operate ancillary equipment such as cranes, fork-lift trucks, etc. (T)
- Operate in a pressurised suit environment. (T)

**The *decommissioning operator* will understand:**
- Routine decommissioning activities. (T)
- Minimisation, packaging and removal of hazardous materials and their transfer to designated storage areas. (T)

**The *decommissioning operator* will understand:**
- The safety, security and behavioural expectations of those working on a nuclear site. (R)
- The fundamental principles of and implications of radiation hazards. (R, T)
- The procedures for dealing with radioactive discharges, waste, environmental control and emergencies. (R)
- The reasons for and application of a variety of safety management systems such as permit to work, standard operating procedures and risk assessment. (R, T)
- The implications and relevance of company policy, external legislation and regulation on working practices (including environmental control). (R)

**The *decommissioning operator* will be capable in:**
- Communications, numeracy, IT, team working, personal development. (P)

**Additionally, the *decommissioning operator* may be required to:**
- Take responsibility for competing tasks and procedures. (P)
- Work independently subject to overall direction or guidance. (P)
- Contribute to improvement of collaborative working. (P)
- Take responsibility for coaching others where appropriate. (P)
- Take responsibility for personal development. (P)

**The *decommissioning operator* may be required to:**
- Solve routine problems using efficiency improvement techniques. (B)
- Apply workplace organisation techniques. (B)
- Understand the practice associated with a variety of appropriate efficiency improvement techniques. (B)

**Advised training/CPD** — Technical (T), Regulatory (R), Business (B), Personal (P)

- Nuclear decommissioning fundamentals. (T)
- Nuclear security, safety and safety culture. (T, R)
- Basic nuclear industry awareness, context and behaviours. (R)
- Safety health and environmental legislation. (R)
- Safety management systems (R, T)
- Radiological protection (T, R)
- Job-related policies and procedures. (T, R, B)
- Industrial safety. (B)

| Nuclear maintenance fitter (mechanical, electrical, instrumentation) | |
|---|---|
| **Sector:** NPP – Decommissioning | |
| **Function:** NPP-D/Maintenance | |
| **Occupational level:** Craft | |
| **Nuclearisation:** *** | |
| **Job title** | **Entry level qualification** |
| **Nuclear maintenance fitter** (mechanical, electrical, instrumentation) | School leaving certificates. |

**Job descriptor**

The *nuclear maintenance fitter* is part of a team preparing work areas for maintenance and reinstating the area upon completion. Capable of conducting planned maintenance activities within their area of specialism (mechanical, electrical or control and instrumentation).

**Competencies** — Technical (T), Regulatory (R), Business (B), Personal (P)

**The *nuclear maintenance fitter* will be able to:**
- Prepare work area for maintenance of plant, systems or components. (T)
- Carry out planned maintenance activities efficiently. (T)
- Reinstate work area after completion of maintenance of plant, systems or components. (T)
- Conduct safe and effective handover of plant and equipment and accept and confirm responsibility for the control of the plant and equipment with the work isolation boundary. (T)
- Identify obsolescence and end-of-life issues. (T)

**The *nuclear maintenance fitter* will understand:**
- How to read and extract information from engineering drawings, specification diagrams and maintenance manuals. (T)
- Technical details relating to the individual's specialist discipline (mechanical/electrical/instrumentation). (T)

**The *nuclear maintenance fitter* will understand:**
- Safety, security and behavioural expectations of those working on a nuclear site. (R)
- Fundamental principles of and implications of radiation hazards. (R, T)
- Procedures for dealing with radioactive discharges, waste, environmental control and emergencies. (R)
- Reasons for and application of a variety of safety management systems, such as permit to work, standard maintenance procedures and point of work risk assessment. (R, T)
- Implications and relevance of company policy, external legislation and regulation on working practices (including environmental control). (R)

***The nuclear maintenance fitter* will be capable in:**
- Basic communications. (P)
- Numeracy. (P)
- IT. (P)
- Team working. (P)
- Personal development. (P)

**The *nuclear maintenance fitter* may be required to:**
- Take responsibility for competing tasks and procedures. (P)
- Work independently subject to overall direction or guidance. (P)
- Contribute to improvement of collaborative working. (P, B)
- Take responsibility for coaching others where appropriate. (P)
- Take responsibility for personal development. (P)

**The *nuclear maintenance fitter* may be required to:**
- Solve routine problems using efficiency improvement techniques. (B)
- Apply workplace organisation techniques. (B)
- Understand the practice associated with a variety of appropriate efficiency improvement techniques. (B)

**Advised training/CPD** — Technical (T), Regulatory (R), Business (B), Personal (P)

- Licensed to practice engineering in the applicable jurisdiction. (T, R)
- Engineering maintenance. (T)
- Business improvement. (B)
- Nuclear security, safety and safety culture. (T, R)
- Job-related policies and procedures. (T, R, B)
- Nuclear industry induction, context, behaviours. (R)
- Nuclear security, safety and safety culture. (T, R)
- Safety, health and environmental regulation. (T, R)
- Vocational courses as appropriate. (T, R, P)
- Supervisor training. (P)

| **Radioactive waste operations manager** | |
|---|---|
| **Sector:** | **NPP – Decommissioning** |
| **Function:** | **NPP-D/Waste management** |
| **Occupational level:** | **Professional** |
| **Nuclearisation:** | *** |

| **Job title** | **Entry level qualification** |
|---|---|
| **Radioactive waste operations manager** | Degree or equivalent vocational qualification with suitable experience. |

**Job descriptor**

The *radioactive waste operations manager* allocates personnel to carry out radioactive waste operations, monitors implementation of plans and procedures to ensure compliance with project schedules, safety procedures and legislation. Controls and develops plans and procedures and resolves problems arising during radioactive waste management activities.

**Competencies** — Technical (T), Regulatory (R), Business (B), Personal (P)

**The *radioactive waste operations manager* will be able to:**

- Control and develop plans and procedures. (T)
- Allocate personnel to prepare for/carry out radioactive waste operations. (T)
- Respond to and solve radioactive waste operational problems. (T)
- Monitor implementation of plans and procedures to ensure compliance with project schedules, safety procedures and legislation. (T, R)

**The *radioactive waste operations manager* will understand:**

- Practice involved with the optimisation, packaging and removal of hazardous materials and their transfer to designated storage areas. (T, R)
- Radioactivity and nuclear science and engineering. (T)
- Methods of radioactive waste characterisation. (T)
- How to fix high activity, mobile contamination. (T)
- How to use maths, IT and problem solving techniques. (T)

**The *radioactive waste operations manager* will understand:**

- Safety, security and behavioural expectations of those working on nuclear sites. (R)
- Fundamental principles and implications of radiation hazards. (R, T)
- Construction of and standards used in a modern standards nuclear safety case. (R)
- Procedures for dealing with radioactive discharges, waste, environmental control and emergencies. (R)
- Reasons for and application of a variety of safety management systems such as permit to work, standard operating procedures and risk assessment. (R, T)
- Implications and relevance of company policy, external legislation and regulation on working practices (including environmental control). (R)
- His/her responsibilities for controlling workplace hazards and managing the health and safety of others. (R)
- Personal responsibilities to ensure compliance with legal, regulatory, ethical and social requirements. (R)

***The radioactive waste operations manager* will have the ability to:**

- Develop and maintain productive working relationships with colleagues and stakeholders. (P)
- Provide learning opportunities for colleagues. (P)
- Manage his/her professional development by setting targets and planning how they will be met. (P)
- Put across ideas in clear and concise manner and present a well structured case. (P)
- Communicate complex information to others. (P)
- Handover at end of shift. (P)

**The *radioactive waste operations manager* may be required to:**

- Understand the theory, principles and practice associated with a variety of appropriate business improvement techniques. (B)
- Solve process problems using business improvement techniques. (B)
- Encourage innovation within his/her team. (B)
- Implement quality assurance systems. (B)

**Advised training/CPD** — Technical (T), Regulatory (R), Business (B), Personal (P)

- Science and engineering of nuclear decommissioning. (T)
- Science of ionising radiation. (T)
- Radiological protection. (T, R)
- Business improvement techniques. (B)
- Risk assessment and management. (B, T)
- Nuclear industry induction, awareness and behaviours. (R)
- Nuclear regulation compliance. (R)
- Safety, health and environmental legislation. (R)
- Leadership and management. (P)
- Nuclear security, safety and safety culture. (T, R)
- Job-related policies and procedures. (T, R, B)

## Radioactive waste supervisor

**Sector:** NPP – Decommissioning
**Function:** NPP-D/Waste management
**Occupational level:** Technical
**Nuclearisation:** ***

| Job title | Entry level qualification |
|---|---|
| **Radioactive waste supervisor** also known as **radioactive waste operations team leader** | Vocational qualification (technical area). |

**Job descriptor**

The *radioactive waste supervisor* is responsible for the safe and efficient management of a team undertaking radioactive waste management activities within the scope of their authority. Ensures that health and safety legislative requirements are adhered to.

**Competencies** — Technical (T), Regulatory (R), Business (B), Personal (P)

**The *radioactive waste supervisor* will be able to:**
- Demonstrate a thorough understanding of radioactive waste management practices. (T)
- Take a leading role in contributing ideas for the control and implementation of work. (T)
- Allocate effectively and fairly work to the radioactive waste operations team and supervise radiation related work activities. (T, P)
- Manage a team delivering a radioactive waste operation, ensuring that key objectives are achieved. (T, P)
- Implement safe access systems in a radiation/contamination controlled environment. (T, R)
- Enable learning within the decommissioning team through demonstration, instruction and coaching. (T, P)

**The *radioactive waste supervisor* will understand:**
- The practice involved in carrying out routine radioactive waste management activities within the nuclear industry. (T, R)
- The practice involved with the minimisation, packaging and removal of hazardous materials and transfer of materials to designated storage area. (T, R)

**The *radioactive waste supervisor* will understand:**
- The safety, security and behavioural expectations of those working on a nuclear site. (R)
- The fundamental principles and implications of radiation hazards. (R, T)
- The procedures for dealing with radioactive discharges, waste, environmental control and emergencies. (R)
- The reasons for and application of a variety of safety management systems such as permit to work, standard operating procedures and risk assessment. (R, T)
- The implications and relevance of company policy, external legislation and regulation on working practices (including environmental control). (R)

**The *radioactive waste supervisor* will be capable in/can:**
- Basic skills in communications, numeracy and IT. (P)
- Take responsibility for completing tasks and procedures. (P)
- Exercise autonomy and judgment subject to overall direction or guidance. (P)
- Develop co-operative relationships with others. (P)
- Plan work with others and review progress against objectives. (P)
- Contribute towards the improvement of collaborative working. (P)
- Take responsibility for supervising or guiding others where appropriate. (P)
- Take responsibility for personal development by setting targets and planning how they will be met. (P)
- Review progress towards targets and establish evidence of achievements. (P)
- Communicate complex information to others. (P)
- Handover at end of shift. (P)

**The *radioactive waste supervisor* may be required to:**
- Apply a variety of appropriate business improvement techniques to solve business problems and improve business efficiency. (B)
- Solve routine operational problems using business improvement techniques. (B)
- Understand the theory principles and practice associated with a variety of appropriate business improvement techniques. (B)

**Advised training/CPD** — Technical (T), Regulatory (R), Business (B), Personal (P)

- Nuclear industry induction, awareness and behaviours. (R)
- Nuclear regulation compliance. (R)
- Radiological protection and regulation. (T, R)
- Safety, health and environmental legislation. (R)
- Safety management systems. (R)
- Nuclear security, safety and safety culture. (T, R)
- Leadership and management. (P)
- Radioactive waste management and regulation. (T, R)
- Job-related policies and procedures. (T, R, B)
- Fundamentals of ionising radiation. (T)
- Business improvement techniques. (B)
- Risk assessment and management. (B, T)

## Radiation protection team leader

**Sector:** NPP – Decommissioning
**Function:** NPP-D/Safety and environment
**Occupational level:** Technical
**Nuclearisation:** ***

| Job title | Entry level qualification |
|---|---|
| **Radiation protection team leader**, also known as **radiation protection supervisor** and **health physics foreman** | Vocational qualification with appropriate experience. |

**Job descriptor**

The *radiation protection team leader* identifies and quantifies radiation hazards. Supervises radiation protection monitoring activities. Capable of undertaking all of the tasks conducted by their monitors/surveyors and of delivering the organisations radiation protection service to defined standards.

**Competencies** — Technical (T), Regulatory (R), Business (B), Personal (P)

**The *radiation protection team leader* will be able to:**
- Deliver a radiation protection monitoring service to defined standards. (T, R)
- Identify and quantify radiation hazards and supervise radiation protection monitoring activities. (T)
- Conduct radiation protection monitoring. (T)
- Respond to changes in radiological conditions. (T)
- Deliver radiation protection training. (T, P)

**The *radiation protection team leader* additionally may be required to:**
- Assess, authorise and assign colleagues to undertake radiation-related work. (T, P)
- Manage information on radiation protection and participate in site emergency response arrangements. (T, R, P)
- Prepare and report against risk assessments procedures and instructions. (T, R)

**The *radiation protection team leader* will understand:**
- Fundamental principles and implications of radiation types, sources, hazards and appropriate control measures. (T)
- Purpose and limitations of different types of radiation protection monitoring equipment. (T)
- Principles of designating supervised and controlled areas. (T, R)

**The *radiation protection team leader* will be capable in:**
- Communications, numeracy, IT, team working, personal development. (P)
- Responsibility for competing tasks and procedures. (P)
- Independent working subject to overall direction or guidance. (P)
- Developing co-operative relationships with others. (P)
- Planning work with others and review progress against objectives. (P)
- Contributing to improvement of collaborative working. (P)
- Responsibility for supervising or guiding others where appropriate. (P)
- Responsibility for personal development by setting targets and planning how they will be met. (P)
- Reviewing progress towards targets and establish evidence of achievements. (P)
- Handover at end of shift. (P)

**The *radiation protection team leader* will understand:**
- Safety, security and behavioural expectations of those working on a nuclear site. (R)
- Fundamental principles of and implications of radiation hazards. (R, T)
- Procedures for dealing with radioactive discharges, waste, environmental control and emergency. (R)
  Reasons for and application of a variety of safety management systems such as permit to work, standard operating procedures and risk assessment. (R, T)
- Significance and relevance of company policy, ionising radiation regulations and other legislation and regulation, on working practices (including environmental control). (R)

**The *radiation protection team leader* may be required to:**
- Understand the theory, principles and practice associated with a variety of appropriate business improvement techniques. (B)
- Solve process problems using business improvement techniques. (B)

**Advised training/CPD** — Technical (T), Regulatory (R), Business (B), Personal (P)

- Science of radiation. (T)
- Radiological protection (advanced). (T)
- Business improvement techniques. (B)
- Risk assessment and management. (B, T)
- Nuclear security, safety and safety culture. (T, R)
- Nuclear industry awareness, context, behaviours, regulations. (R)
- Safety, health and environmental legislation. (R)
- Nuclear regulation compliance. (R)
- Radiological regulation (advanced). (R)
- Leadership and management. (P)
- Job-related policies and procedures. (T, R, B)

| Radiation protection health physics surveyor | |
|---|---|
| **Sector:** NPP – Decommissioning<br>**Function:** NPP – D/Safety and environment<br>**Occupational level:** Craft<br>**Nuclearisation:** *** | |
| **Job title** | **Entry level qualification** |
| **Radiation protection health physics surveyor** | Vocational qualification with appropriate experience. |

**Job descriptor**

The *radiation protection health physics surveyor* undertakes monitoring for personnel, surface and airborne contamination levels and dose rates. Records the levels detected and responds according. May also undertake radiation-related work activities and be part of the emergency response arrangements.

**Competencies** — Technical (T), Regulatory (R), Business (B), Personal (P)

**The *radiation protection health physics surveyor* will be able to:**
- Monitor surface and airborne contamination and respond accordingly. (T)
- Monitor radiation dose rate levels and respond accordingly. (T)
- Monitor personnel for surface contamination and respond accordingly. (T)
- Undertake clearance monitoring. (T)
- Function test radiation protection monitoring equipment. (T)
- Respond to changes in radiological conditions. (T)
- Record radiation protection monitoring and survey results. (T)

**The *radiation protection health physics surveyor* may be required to:**
- Undertake radiation-related work activities. (T)
- Participate in site emergency response arrangements. (T)
- Collect and process radioactive solid waste. (T)

**The *radiation protection health physics surveyor* will understand:**
- The fundamental principles and implications of radiation types, sources, hazards and appropriate control measures. (T, r)
- The purpose and limitations of different types of radiation protection monitoring equipment. (T)

**The *radiation protection health physics surveyor* may be required to:**
- Solve routine problems using efficiency improvement techniques. (B)
- Apply workplace organisation techniques. (B)
- Understand the practice associated with a variety of appropriate efficiency improvement techniques. (B)

**The *radiation protection health physics surveyor* will understand:**
- The safety, security and behavioural expectations of those working on a nuclear site. (R)
- The procedures for dealing with radioactive discharges, waste, environmental control and emergency procedures. (R)
- The reasons for and application of a variety of safety management systems such as permit to work, standard operating procedures and risk assessment. (R, t)
- The significance and relevance of company policy, ionising radiation regulations and other legislation and regulation, on working practices (including environmental control). (R)

**The *radiation protection health physics surveyor* will be capable in:**
- Communications, numeracy, IT, team working, personal development. (P)

**The *radiation protection health physics surveyor* may:**
- Take responsibility for competing tasks and procedures. (P)
- Work independently subject to overall direction or guidance. (P)
- Contribute to improvement of collaborative working. (P)
- Take responsibility for coaching others where appropriate. (P)
- Take responsibility for personal development. (P)

**Advised training/CPD** — Technical (T), Regulatory (R), Business (B), Personal (P)

- Nuclear industry induction, context, behaviours and regulations. (R)
- Fundamentals of radiation. (T)
- Radiological protection and regulation. (T, R)
- Nuclear security, safety and safety culture. (T, R)
- Safety, health and environmental legislation. (R)
- Risk assessment and management. (B, T)
- Business improvement techniques. (B)
- Nuclear regulation compliance. (R)
- Job-related practices and procedures. (T, R, B)
- Supervisor training. (P)


NUCLEAR EDUCATION AND TRAINING: FROM CONCERN TO CAPABILITY, ISBN 978-92-64-17637-9, © OECD 2012

| Safety case lead author | |
|---|---|
| **Sector:** NPP – Decommissioning<br>**Function:** NPP-D/Safety and environment<br>**Occupational level:** Professional<br>**Nuclearisation:** *** | |
| **Job title** | **Entry level qualification** |
| **Safety case lead author** | Degree in relevant science engineering or technology, or vocational qualification with suitable experience. |

**Job descriptor**

The *safety case lead author* brings together elements of the safety case to provide clear and concise safety arguments to form a "fit for purpose" safety case. The *lead author* will be responsible for bringing together delivery of the safety case. The *lead author* may be supported by less experienced personnel such as: a *competent safety case author* who provides unsupervised support to the lead author, also *junior safety case authors* who provide supervised support to the *lead author.*

**Competencies** — Technical (T), Regulatory (R), Business (B), Personal (P)

**The *safety case lead author* will be able to:**

- Produce nuclear safety cases in accordance with organisational procedures including (T, B):
- Liaise with stakeholders involved. (T, P)
- Obtain contextual information. (T, P)
- Identify safety hazards using complementary techniques. (T)
- Develop safety claims for use in nuclear safety cases. (T)
- Articulat ideas and write arguments and technical content in a clear and concise manner, presenting a well structured case. (T, P)
- Commission the production of evidence. (T)
- Provide risk assessments including identification of engineering and administrative controls from the safety case which can be implemented within the plant. (T)
- Verify evidence. (T)
- Manage the review and approval of safety cases. (T)
- Support "due process" requirements. (T)
- Support through-life safety issues, including periodic review, optioneering reviews and plant modifications. (T)
- Provide information and advice. (T)

**The *safety case lead author* additionally may be required to:**

- Plan and co-ordinate the preparation of nuclear safety cases. (T, P)
- Assist the safety case officer establish the scope and strategy for the production/development of nuclear safety cases. (T)

**The *safety case lead author* will understand:**

- Structure of modern standards for nuclear safety cases, including deterministic and probabilistic safety assessment and engineering substantiation. (T, R)
- Requirements of nuclear safety case "due process". (T)
- ALARP (as low as reasonably practicable) principle and its application throughout the safety case lifecycle. (T, R)
- Engineering design and operation of the plant/equipment being assessed. (T)
- How the safety case can be implemented and how it integrates with the design and operation of the plant/equipment being assessed. (T)
- Safety case standards and methodologies. (T, R)
- Radiological consequences and regulatory limits of exposures to radiation. (T, R)
- Need for specialist subject analysis. (T)

**The *safety case lead author* will understand:**

- Safety, security and behavioural expectations of those working on a nuclear site. (R, P)
- Fundamental principles of and implications of radiation hazards. (R, T)
- Procedures for dealing with radioactive discharges, waste, environmental control and emergencies. (R)
- Reasons for and application of a variety of safety management systems such as permit to work, standard operating & maintenance procedures and risk assessment. (R)
- Implications and relevance of company policy, external legislation and regulation on working practices (including environmental control). (R, T)
- The responsibilities for controlling workplace hazards and managing the health and safety of others. (R)
- The responsibilities to comply with legal, regulatory, ethical and social requirements. (R)

***The safety case lead author* will be capable in:**

- Developing and maintaining productive working relationships with colleagues and stakeholders. (P)
- Providing learning opportunities for colleagues. (P)
- Managing professional development by setting targets and planning how they will be met. (P)
- Communicating complex information to others. (P)
- Mentoring less experienced/junior safety case authors. (P)

**The *safety case lead author* may be required to:**

- Understand the theory, principles and practice associated with a variety of appropriate business improvement techniques. (B)
- Solve process problems using business improvement techniques. (B)
- Encourage innovation within his/her team. (B)
- Implement quality assurance systems. (B)

| Advised training/CPD | Technical (T), Regulatory (R), Business (B), Personal (P) |
|---|---|
| – Nuclear plant design. (T)<br>– Science and engineering of nuclear decommissioning. (T)<br>– Safety case specialisms. (T)<br>– Radiological protection (advanced). (T, R)<br>– Business improvement techniques. (B)<br>– Risk assessment and management. (B, T) | – Nuclear industry awareness, behaviours and context. (R)<br>– Nuclear security, safety and safety culture. (T, R)<br>– Safety, health and environmental legislation (advanced). (R)<br>– National and international guidelines and legislation and regulations as appropriation. (R)<br>– Radiological regulation (advanced). (R)<br>– Job-related policy and regulation procedures and practice (advanced). (T, B, R)<br>– Leadership and management. (P) |

## Table A4.8: Job profiles for nuclear research reactors

### Reactor manager

**Sector:** NRR
**Function:** NRR/Operation and control
**Occupational level:** Professional
**Nuclearisation:** ***

| Job title | Entry level qualification |
|---|---|
| Reactor manager | Master degree in engineering with several years nuclear training and experience in commissioning, maintenance or operation of a nuclear power plant, test reactor, research reactor or production reactor, or a critical facility. |

**Job descriptor**

The *reactor manager* has direct responsibility for all aspects of the operation, utilisation and modification of the reactor. In discharging this responsibility, the *reactor manager* should also be responsible for the overall co-ordination of technical support functions. The *reactor manager* is responsible for the qualification (including adequate initial training and continuing training) of the operating personnel.

**Competencies** — Technical (T), Regulatory (R), Business (B), Personal (P)

**The *reactor manager* will:**
- Be responsible for the safety of all operations under his control. (T)
- Establish operational performance standards and management expectations for all activities relating to safe operation and utilisation of the reactor and effectively communicate these standards throughout the operating organisation. (T, R, P)
- Set operational performance standards and expectations for the operating personnel in all aspects of the safe management of the reactor. (T, R)
- Ensure that personnel are aware of and accept their responsibilities for maintaining a high level of safety. (T, B)
- Ensure compliance with the requirements of the operating organisation and the regulatory body. (T, R)
- Manage the scientific programme of the reactor.(T)
- Recognise, and help to meet, the need to develop the managerial and technical skills of all individuals involved in activities relating to the reactor facility. (T, B)
- Submit periodic summary reports on matters relating to safety to the safety committee for its consideration and should consider any information provided in response. (T, R)

**The *reactor manager* will understand:**
- The safety, security and behavioural expectations of those working on nuclear sites. (R)
- The fundamental principles of reactor operations. (R, T)
- The fundamental principles and implications of radiation hazards. (R, T)
- The reasons for and application of a variety of safety management systems. (R)
- The implications and relevance of company policy, external legislation and regulation on working practices. (R)

**The *reactor manager* can:**
- Demonstrate excellent management and leadership skills including management of personnel, planning and budget. (P)
- Effectively manage crises. (P)
- Demonstrate strong analytical and problem solving skills. (P)
- Communicate complex information in a clear and concise manner. (P)
- Develop and maintain productive working relationships with colleagues and stakeholders. (P)
- Provide learning opportunities for colleagues. (P)
- Manage professional development by setting targets and planning how they will be met. (P)

**The *reactor manager* may be required to:**
- Understand the theory, principles and practise associated with a variety of appropriate business improvement techniques. (B)
- Solve operational problems using business improvement techniques. (B)
- Encourage innovation within his/her team. (B)
- Implement quality assurance systems. (B)

**Advised training/CPD** — Technical (T), Regulatory (R), Business (B), Personal (P)

- Nuclear security, safety and safety culture. (T, R)
- On the job training at a research reactor facility may qualify as equivalent nuclear experience (from IAEA NS-G-4.5). (T)
- Radiation protection and regulation (advanced). (T, R)
- Statutory bases: national and international regulations. (R, T)
- Facility engineering. (T)
- Facility operation. (T)
- Administrative requirements (management, communication). (P)
- Internal training in company procedures with respect to business practises. (B)
- Nuclear security, safety and safety culture. (T, R)
- Nuclear industry awareness, context and behaviours. (T, R)
- Safety, health and environmental legislation (advanced). (R)
- Safety management systems. (T, R)
- National and international guidelines and legislation and regulations as appropriation. (R)
- Radiological regulation. (R)
- Policy and regulation procedures and practice (advanced). (R)
- Risk assessment. (T, R)
- National and international guidelines and legislation and regulations as appropriation. (R)
- Job-related policy and regulation procedures and practice (advanced). (T, R, B)
- Leadership and management. (P)

## Reactor operator

**Sector:** NRR
**Function:** Operation and control
**Occupational level:** Technical
**Nuclearisation:** ***

| Job title | Entry level qualification |
|---|---|
| **Reactor operator** | Secondary technical education. |

**Job descriptor**

The *reactor operator* is in charge of operating the reactor. This will include loading/unloading of the reactors, providing technical support for the maintenance as well as the administrative tasks inherent in the operation of the reactors.

**Competencies** — Technical (T), Regulatory (R), Business (B), Personal (P)

**The *reactor operator* will be able to:**
- Take the necessary measures to start, operate and shut down the reactor and corresponding instrumentation. (T)
- Have the authority and responsibility to shut down the reactor if necessary for safety purposes. (T)
- Control all parameters of the reactor's nuclear and conventional circuits and corresponding instrumentation. (T)
- Realise specific radiation experiments. (T)
- Manage experimental data using computer programs. (T)
- Perform periodic inspections of the controlled area and act conform facility procedures on abnormal phenomena. (T, R)
- Take prescript measures in case of emergency. (T, R)
- Give technical support during maintenance works on the reactor and its installations. (T)
- Keep up-to-date knowledge about the operation of the reactor and its installations. (T)

**The *reactor operator* will understand:**
- The safety, security and behavioural expectations of those working on nuclear sites. (R)
- The fundamental principles of reactor operations. (R, T)
- The fundamental principles and implications of radiation hazards. (R, T)
- The reasons for and application of a variety of safety management systems. (R)
- The implications and relevance of company policy, external legislation and regulation on working practices. (R)

**The *reactor operator* will be capable in/can:**
- Basic skills in communication, numeracy and IT. (P)
- Take responsibility for completing tasks and procedures. (P)
- Develop co-operative relationships with others. (P)
- Exercise autonomy and judgement subject to overall direction or guidance. (P)
- Planning and organisation skills. (P)
- Manage his/her personal development by setting targets and planning how they will be met. (P)
- Plan work with others and review progress against objectives. (P)
- Handover at end of shift. (P)

**The *reactor operator* may be required to:**
- Understand the theory, principles and practice associated with a variety of appropriate business improvement techniques. (B)
- Solve operational problems using business improvement techniques. (B)

**Advised training/CPD** — Technical (T), Regulatory (R), Business (B), Personal (P)

- Secondary technical. (T)
- Accreditation given after at least two years of nuclear experience and training:
  - nuclear physics. (T)
  - reactor physics. (T)
  - reactor safety. (T, R)
  - radiation protection. (T, R)
  - facility engineering (reactor auxiliary systems). (T)
  - occupational safety. (T, R)
- Internal training in company procedures with respect to business practices. (B)
- Nuclear security, safety and safety culture. (T, R)
- Nuclear industry awareness, context and behaviours. (T, R)
- Safety, health and environmental legislation (advanced). (R)
- Safety management systems. (T, R)
- National and international guidelines and legislation and regulations as appropriation. (R)
- Radiological regulation. (R)
- Policy and regulation procedures and practice (advanced). (R)
- Leadership and management. (P)

| **Radiation protection officer** | |
|---|---|
| **Sector:** | **NRR** |
| **Function:** | **Operation and control** |
| **Occupational level:** | **Technical** |
| **Nuclearisation:** | *** |

| **Job title** | **Entry level qualification** |
|---|---|
| **Radiation protection officer** | Secondary technical education in electronics, electro-mechanics or industrial sciences. |

**Job descriptor**

The *radiation protection officer* is an individual who is technically competent in matters of radiation protection relevant to the research reactor facility and who is designated by the operating organisation to oversee the application of the requirements for radiation protection. One of the *radiation protection officer's* main responsibilities is to prepare and conduct the radiation protection programme.

**Competencies** — Technical (T), Regulatory (R), Business (B), Personal (P)

**The *radiation protection officer* will be able to:**

- Monitor and measure radiation and/or contamination levels for personnel, rooms and objects. (T)
- Provide expert advice and assistance to the facility management in specifying and carrying out its responsibilities for the radiation protection programme. (T, R)
- Review for approval, in accordance with established policy, all procedures, work practices, radiation protection manuals, equipment, proposed changes to the design of the facility, training programmes and reactor experiments, as they pertain to radiation protection. (T, R, B)
- Provide expert advice on and assistance in matters of radiation protection to facility staff. (T, R, B)
- Assess the effectiveness and efficiency of all aspects of the facility operations relating to radiation protection. (T)
- Provide radiation protection services in accordance with the policy of the management and the needs of the facility. (T, B)
- Guide and oversee the application of the optimisation (ALARA) principle. (T, R)
- Implement an internal programme of review and verification (e.g. audits) to ensure that approved procedures relating to radiation protection have been documented and are carried out accordingly. (T, B)
- Initiate corrective actions when deviations from approved procedures are observed. (T, B)
- Provide first-aid care when necessary. (T)

**The *radiation protection officer* will understand:**

- The safety, security and behavioural expectations of those working on nuclear sites. (R)
- The fundamental principles and implications of radiation hazards. (R, T)
- The reasons for and application of a variety of safety management systems. (R)
- The procedures for dealing with radioactive discharges, waste, environmental control and emergency procedures. (R)
- The implications and relevance of company policy, external legislation and regulation on working practices (including environmental control). (R)

**The *radiation protection officer* will be capable in/can:**

- Communication, numeracy and IT. (P)
- Take responsibility for completing tasks and procedures. (P)
- Develop co-operative relationships with others. (P)
- Work independently subject to overall direction or guidance. (P)
- Plan work with others and review progress against objectives. (P )
- Take responsibility for supervising or guiding others when appropriate. (P)
- Manage his/her personal development by setting targets and planning how they will be met. (P)

**The *radiation protection officer* may be required to:**

- Understand the theory, principles and practice associated with a variety of appropriate business improvement techniques. (B)
- Solve operational problems using business improvement techniques. (B)

**Advised training/CPD** — Technical (T), Regulatory (R), Business (B), Personal (P)

- Secondary technical education in electronics, electro-mechanics or industrial sciences. (T)
- Internal training:
  - safety procedures. (R,T, B)
  - administrative procedures. (B)
- Radiation protection. (T, R)
- Internal procedures regarding radiation control and contamination. (T, B)
- Internal training in company procedures with respect to business practices. (B)
- Nuclear security, safety and safety culture. (T, R)
- Nuclear industry awareness, context and behaviours. (T, R)
- Safety, health and environmental legislation (advanced). (R)
- Safety management systems. (T, R)
- National and international guidelines and legislation and regulations as appropriation. (R)
- Radiological regulation. (R)
- Policy and regulation procedures and practice (advanced). (R)
- Leadership and management. (P)

# *Appendix 5*
# Applications of the job taxonomy

## A5.1 Nuclear competence development: a national forecasting and standards model[1]

### *Predicting human resource needs for governments and employers*

Employment in many developed economies operates on the supply and demand for skilled people. The supply of general and specialist skills of young people entering the labour market is largely funded (at least initially) by states through the education system, while demand is determined, in this nuclear context, by the investment decisions of the nuclear operators and induced employment in the supply chain. In this regard employment costs will also include appropriate "nuclearisation" of employees for competence, especially the technical and the regulatory, that are often at the core of compliance.

Both governments and employers can benefit from access to high quality labour market intelligence and training standards. This can inform, for example, targeted policy interventions such as directives on training, or prioritisation on resourcing of higher education and research. For employers, HR development and accreditation can be quality assured through independently verified standards, and accreditation can inform the choice of training, be it in-company, public or private provision.

Figure A5.1 illustrates how the nuclear taxonomy has worked with government scenarios on future "energy pathways" in the United Kingdom. Figure A5.1a indicates a "balanced" low-carbon energy mix with nuclear contributing one-third of supply. Figure A5.1b as reported in the *Next Generation* publication (Cogent, 2010) is derived from a quantitative taxonomy and relates to 16 GWe of new nuclear capacity by 2025 in line with the energy pathway analysis.

### *Quantifying a national labour market for nuclear*

In contrast to the wide range of econometric data collected nationally (e.g. Office for National Statistics, the United Kingdom) and internationally (e.g. Eurostat), there is a paucity of national data on the labour market of the civil nuclear industry. By comparison to, for example, the oil and gas or manufactured fuels industries for which standard industrial and occupational classifications are specified, only the smallest part of the nuclear industry is directly quantified under nuclear fuel processing (as a subset of manufactured fuels). This places great emphasis (in the United Kingdom) on the primary labour market research reported by Cogent, the licensed national skills council for the industry.[2]

Three skills drivers are quantified in the *Power People* report (Cogent, 2009): an ageing workforce driving replacement demand; a short-term shift in skills to decommissioning; and a medium-term demand for skills to build and operate a new fleet of nuclear power stations. Of particular note in this example is the successful collaboration with the industry on a skills classification system – a national nuclear skills taxonomy. The taxonomy has allowed the HR of nuclear to be mapped by region, nation, skill level, age, sub-sector, and job context. Example outputs are given in Figure A5.2.

1. UK model, Cogent Sector Skills Council.
2. www.cogent-ssc.com/research/nuclearresearch.php.

### Figure A5.1: United Kingdom energy pathways and nuclear HR requirements

#### a. Energy pathways

Civil nuclear industry – Job context population 2009

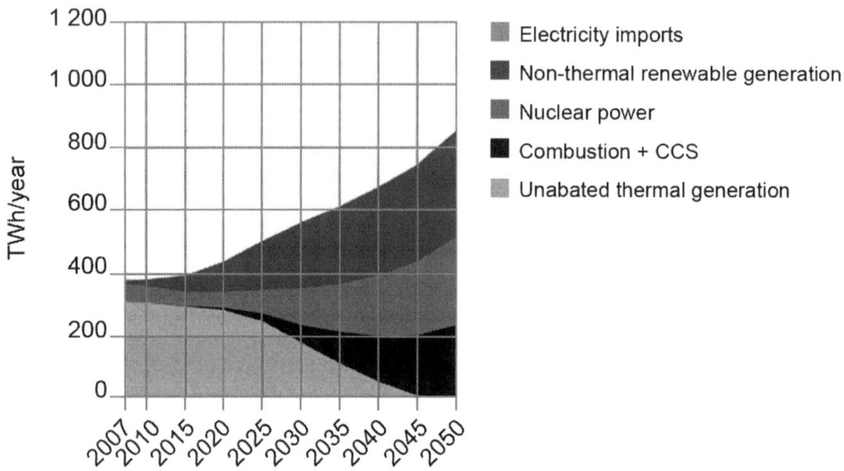


Source: DECC, 2010.

#### b. Nuclear HR requirements

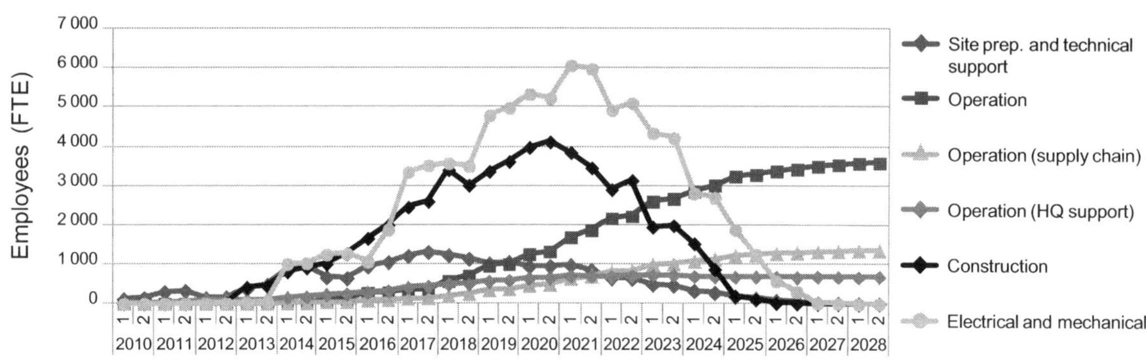


Source: Cogent, 2010.

## Figure A5.2: A national nuclear skills taxonomy (United Kingdom)

### a. Civil nuclear industry by job context

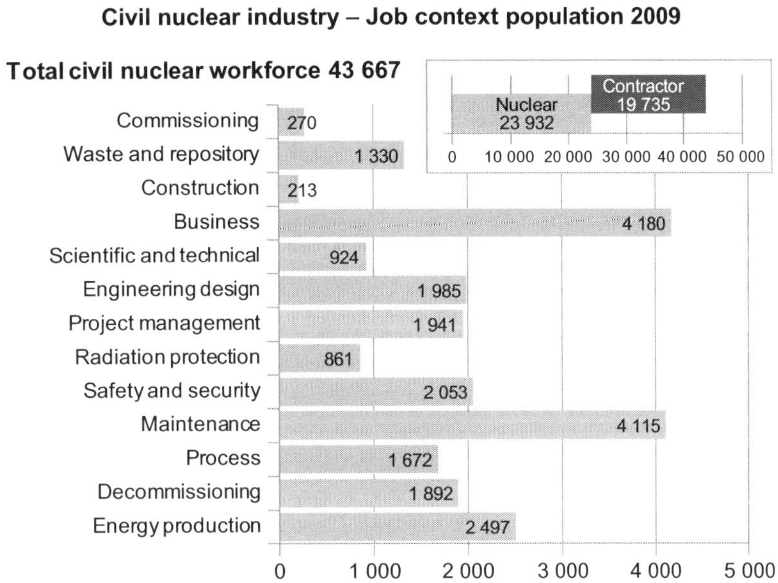


### b. Civil nuclear industry by UK region

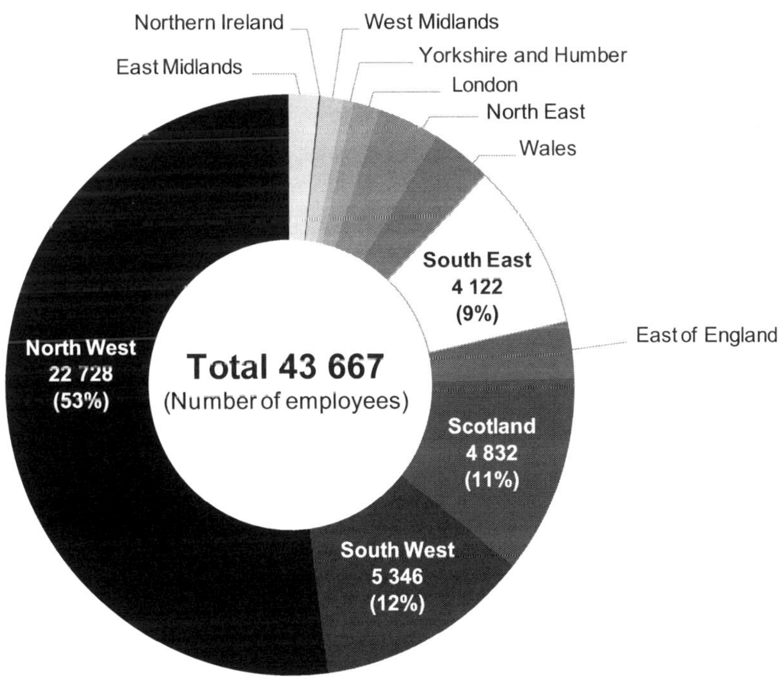


Source: Cogent, 2009.

### *Establishing a nuclear industry training framework, standards and passport*

The Nuclear Industry Training Framework (NITF) encompasses all nuclear job contexts in the United Kingdom, including accredited qualifications and industry standards for a site-licenced company. Shaped with the industry and for the industry, the NITF is the benchmark for employers for skills gap analysis. The nuclear taxonomy underpinned by job contexts provides a common framework for NITF on competencies, qualifications and training. The NITF identifies recognised education and training in four areas: technical, regulatory compliance, business improvement, and functional and behavioural skills.

A key aspect of the NITF is in tracking progress towards a competence profile. This will initially be based on around 13 job contexts in decommissioning operations, energy production operations, process operations, safety and security, etc.

Nuclear Industry Training Standards (NITS) related to these areas have been developed, each with learning outcomes and assessment criteria. The development of these standards has taken place in consultation with the National Skills Academy Nuclear (an accrediting body for training), industry groups and relevant trade, professional or training associations. The NITS provide the quality assurance aspect of the passport.

To date three basic standards have been developed. A similar set will be available soon for people working on new NPP build sites. These must be met by all personnel who will work on a licensed nuclear site. They are:

- basic nuclear industry behaviours;
- basic industry context;
- basic common induction standard.

Founded on the NITF and the NITS is the Nuclear Skills Passport which evidences individual and organisational competence. The passport is underpinned by a database-driven IT platform which provides verification of accredited training. The Nuclear Skills Passport will not carry details of security clearances or act as an identity document to gain site access. Existing site security systems and training on the knowledge of local procedures will remain unchanged.

The Nuclear Skills Passport has been developed with industry consultation to provide the sector with a standardised approach to skills development and recognition, ensuring the strictest security and highest training standards possible. The passport is voluntary but it has been identified by nuclear operators as highly desirable for their supply chain. Figure A5.3 articulates the operational structure of the passport.

The Nuclear Skills Passport will not replace existing nuclear personnel management systems in the short term. However, it will aid licensees, by providing a physical system for proof of skills, in particular for the contractor workforce.

Figure A5.3: **A Nuclear Skills Passport (United Kingdom)**

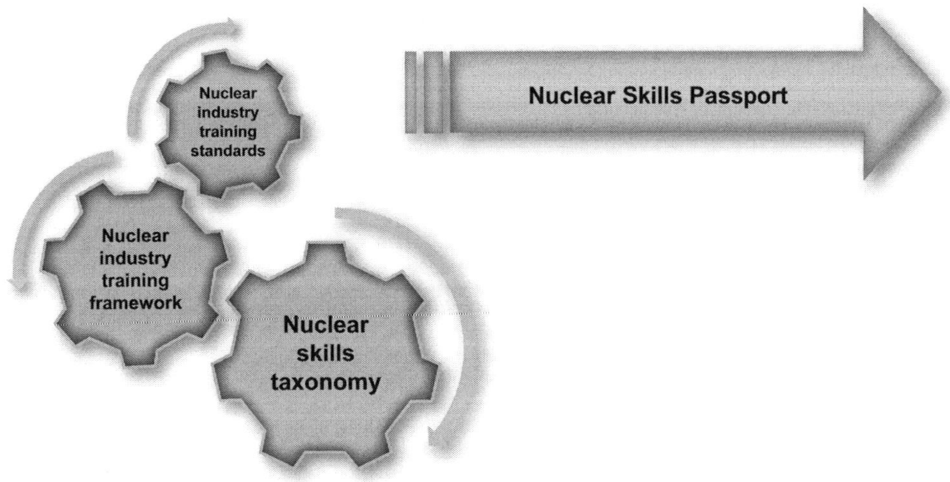


## A5.2 Nuclear competence development: an industrial new build model[3]

### *Overview*

The following paragraphs describe the approach used to formulate an operational preparedness programme for a hypothetical new build by a utility company. The scenario was conceived on the basis of a completely new "greenfield" nuclear programme in a country without any operating plants. The research comprised the development of organisations, infrastructures, facilities and staff recruitment sufficient for the safe operation of two twin PWR sites. The model, as shown below, called for the development of a fully competent organisation of around 1 300 staff to be ready within ten years starting with nothing more than a handful of experienced managers who would, in fact, reach retirement before the completion of the programme.

The process entailed a stepwise approach described in detail below.

### *Determination of a modern best practice organisation*

A process based reference organisation (Figure A5.4) was developed using information from utilities which adopt the Best Practice Standard Nuclear Performance Model (NEI, INPO 1998-2003).

### *Basic educational qualifications, training and experience requirements*

This hypothetical organisation was then developed in detail, down to each of some 200 discrete roles. Each role was then analysed according to competency requirements, from which the related basic educational, training and experience requirements were derived.

Extensive use was made of existing nuclear utility role profile databases in order to cross-check and validate the analysis. No existing structure exactly matched the hypothetical one; nor was it possible to incorporate any regulatory input at this stage. However, the resulting information was judged sufficient to form the basis of a recruitment and development strategy.

3. Prototype kindly provided by David Gilchrist; originally proposed for the Italian nuclear programme.

### *Resource scheduling*

Resource scheduling was planned according to programme milestones, recruitment and training timescales. On the basis of the individual minimum durations for training and experience requirements for each role and the plant construction, licensing and commissioning milestones, it was possible to work back to the recruitment schedule. The resulting aggregate recruitment requirements, categorised by educational qualification, were then determined as shown in Figure A5.5.

The breakdown of aggregate educational requirements including all the construction and engineering resources is shown below. The relative importance of non-nuclear and technical college/ diploma education is often overlooked in the literature and this is underlined by the 50% requirement of diploma-type education. This expertise is typically developed through vocational education and training. The projected figures were:

- Graduates (~ 50%), comprising:
  - nuclear (15%);
  - mechanical (19%);
  - electrical (6%);
  - instrumentation and control (5%);
  - chemistry (2%);
  - civils (2%).
- diploma (50%).

**Figure A5.4: A modern best practice organisation**

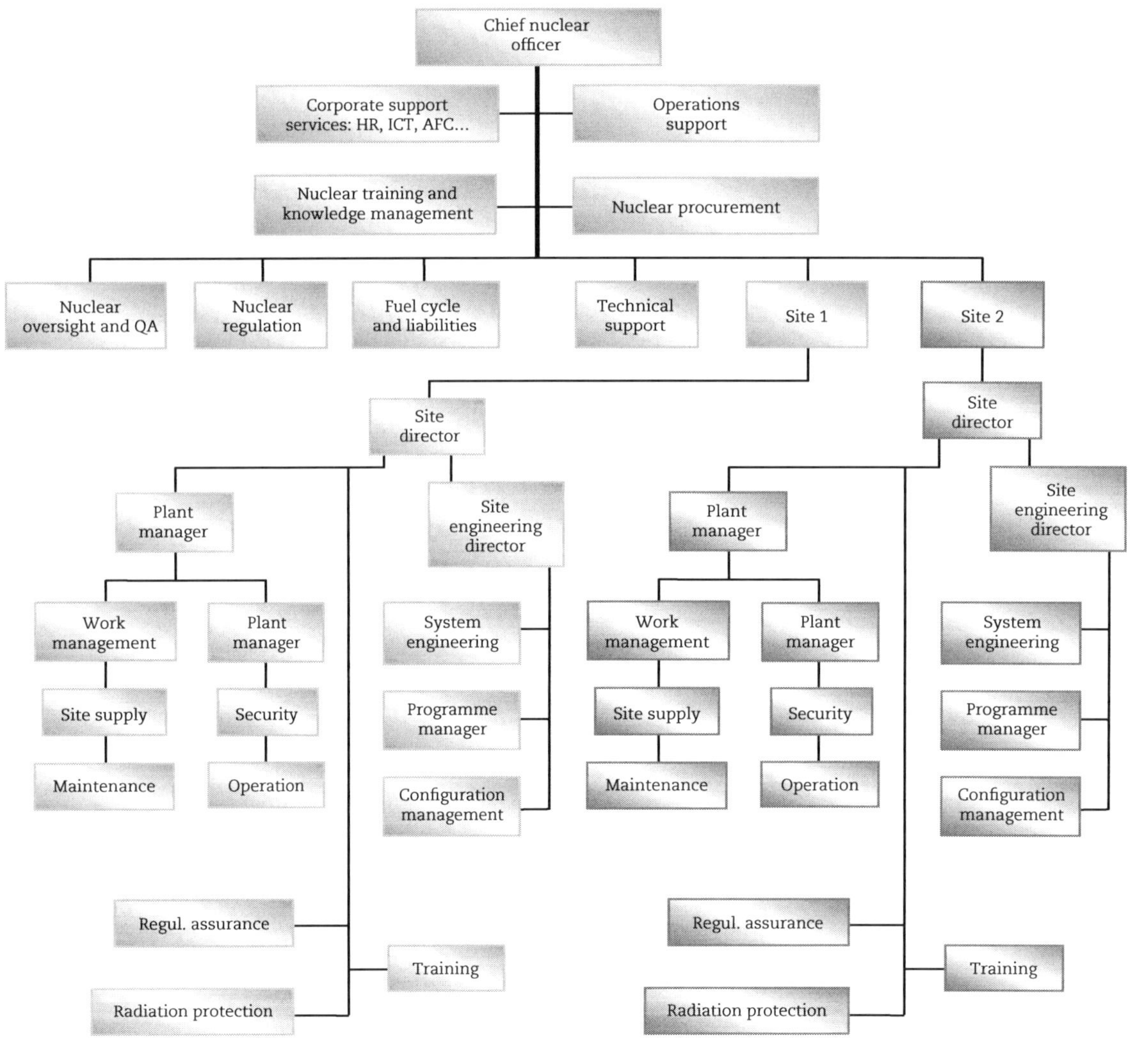


Source: NEI, INPO 1998-2003.



NUCLEAR EDUCATION AND TRAINING: FROM CONCERN TO CAPABILITY, ISBN 978-92-64-17637-9, © OECD 2012

### *Recruitment schedule*

To avoid premature specialisation, recruitment was modelled according to role families. It was felt unproductive at this early stage to set out in precise detail the individual training programmes for each discrete role. The result of this would be a very large series of parallel paths and, in any case, it was deemed impossible to assign individuals to any particular path so many years in advance of their proving their capability (an example rhetorical question to illustrate this would be – *who gets to be site director?*). Instead, the approach adopted to establish the recruitment schedule was to align the roles within job families with common educational and initial training and experience requirements, in other words to generate a job taxonomy that suited the model. This is shown in Figure A5.6.

Figure A5.5: **Resource scheduling – recruitment needs by educational qualifications (excludes construction and central engineering)**

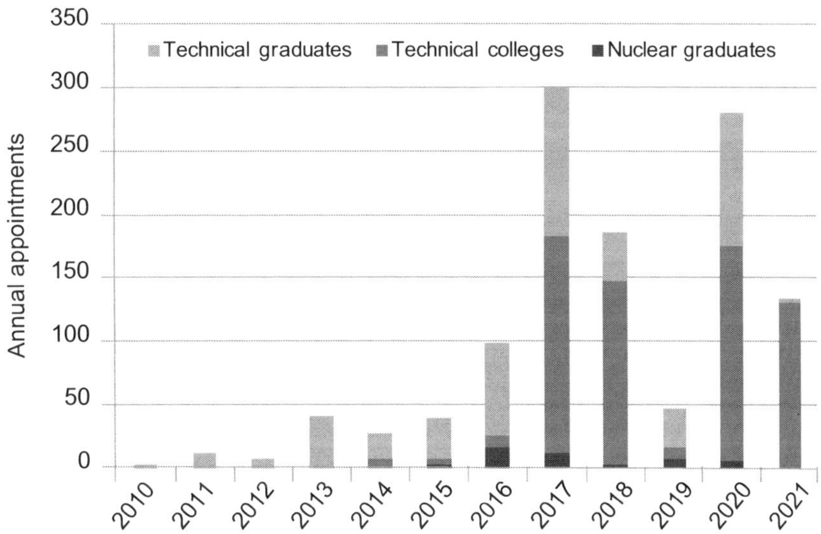


Figure A5.6: **Recruitment schedule**

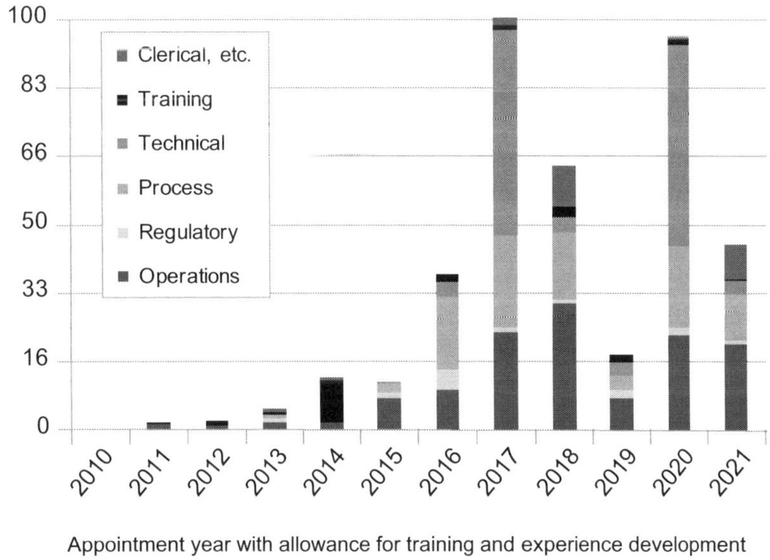

### *Role families and the competence model*

Four principal taxonomic families were established: technical (e.g. engineering), process (e.g. maintenance), regulatory and operations. The defining feature in each case was the dominant competence requirement. A fifth "meta family" – training – was added because of the extraordinary breadth requirements of these roles and the need for their deployment early in the programme. Unsurprisingly, this was deemed the critical path.

It is important to note that competency mapping to taxonomic families was not set as exclusive. The overall scope is similar but the families are differentiated by the degree or depth in a particular competency area. So, for example, all staff had to have a basic "nuclearisation", either through having a nuclear engineering degree or through nuclear induction training. This was then designed to be followed by common programmes on the specific technology, regulatory aspects and, most importantly, nuclear safety culture development.

It is important to note that this approach worked well for the majority of operational, regulatory and process positions but was less useful for the proliferation of technical/specialist engineering roles. The reason for this is their relatively narrow and often unique competence profiles. A civil (seismic) expert, for example, is unlikely to share many competencies with an instrumentation and controls engineer. Consequently the training and development programmes for the engineers tended to diverge from the rest early in the schedule. The challenge then became one of ensuring their continuous engagement in shared fundamental areas such as nuclear safety culture.

### *Infrastructure, leadership and the critical path*

As mentioned previously, the critical path runs through the early establishment of a training infrastructure including competent trainers. It was found to be nearly impossible to find early in the programme any newly recruited staff interested in becoming trainers and, furthermore, the experience duration requirements for certain key roles such as simulator trainer extended beyond the time constraints of the programme. The proposed solution was to re-qualify existing trainers on the new technology in an existing commercial nuclear training organisation. Although not based in the same country, this was feasible for a multinational utility. This facility allowed for the early training for key leadership roles consistent with the overall programme milestones. One such early milestone is the granting of the licence to the licensee who has to fulfil the licence obligations by having a small but nonetheless suitably qualified and experienced organisation well before the plant construction commences. For some of these early key roles, a separate bespoke approach is required – nuclearisation of suitable conventional plant managers is one such possibility.

### *Accreditation strategy*

The accreditation of the licensee training organisation is the next most significant milestone on the operational preparedness programme. No definitive solution was determined; however it was felt important that any solution should have independent accreditation of the training programme. This was deemed necessary to avoid prescriptive regulation in particular, and to avoid the issue of personnel licences by state authorities. In this way the accreditation preserved the principle that the licensee-operator should be uniquely responsible for nuclear safety and also thereby to allow the regulator the freedom to regulate safety through monitoring and inspection rather than administering examinations.

## References

Cogent (2009), *Power People: The Civil Nuclear Workforce 2009-2025*, Renaissance Nuclear Skills Series: 1, Cogent Sector Skills Council, Warrington, United Kingdom, available at: www.cogent-ssc.com/research/renaissance_i.php.

Cogent (2010), *Next Generation Skills for New Build Nuclear*, Renaissance Nuclear Skills Series: 2, Cogent Sector Skills Council, Warrington, United Kingdom, available at: www.cogent-ssc.com/research/nuclearresearch.php.

DECC (2010), *2050 Pathways Analysis*, HM Government, UK, available at: www.decc.gov.uk/assets/decc/what%20we%20do/a%20low%20carbon%20uk/2050/216-2050-pathways-analysis-report.pdf.

# *Appendix 6*
# List of experts

| | |
|---|---|
| **AUSTRALIA** | |
| Ron HUTCHINGS | ANSTO |
| **BELGIUM** | |
| Michel GIOT | SCK•CEN |
| **CANADA** | |
| Basma SHALABY | UNENE |
| **FINLAND** | |
| Kaisa KOSKINEN | Radiation and Nuclear Safety authority (STUK) |
| **FRANCE** | |
| Jean-Philippe NABOT | *Commissariat à l'énergie atomique* (CEA Saclay) |
| **GERMANY** | |
| Xu CHENG | Karlsruher Institute of Technology |
| **ITALY** | |
| Giuliano BUCETI | UTFUS, ENEA |
| **JAPAN** | |
| Hiroyuki MURAKAMI | Japan Atomic Energy Agency |
| **KOREA (REPUBLIC OF)** | |
| Bum-Jin CHUNG | Jeju National University |
| **NETHERLANDS** | |
| Jan Leen KLOOSTERMAN | Delft University of Technology |
| **SPAIN** | |
| Emilio MINGUEZ | Polytechnical University of Madrid (UPM) |
| **SWEDEN** | |
| Jan BLOMGREN | Vattenfall AB |
| **SWITZERLAND** | |
| Rakesh CHAWLA | Paul Scherrer Institute (PSI) |
| **UNITED KINGDOM** | |
| Brian MURPHY | Cogent Sector Skills Council Ltd |
| **UNITED STATES** | |
| Gilbert J. BROWN | University of Massachusetts Lowell |
| Elizabeth MCANDREW-BENAVIDES | Nuclear Energy Institute |
| John GUTTERIDGE | US Nuclear Regulatory Commission |
| Janet GORN | Office of Nuclear Energy, Safety, and Security |
| **European Commission (EC)** | |
| Niina YLIKNUUSSII | Nuclear Fuel Cycle and Waste Administration |
| Georges VAN GOETHEM | Innovation in Nuclear Fission and Education & Training |

**International Atomic Energy Agency (IAEA)**

| | |
|---|---|
| Yanko YANEV | Head Knowledge Mgt Unit, Dept of Nuclear Energy |

**OECD Nuclear Energy Agency (NEA)**

| | |
|---|---|
| Ron CAMERON | Head, Nuclear Development Division (NDD) |
| Maria Elena URSO | Nuclear Analyst, NDD |
| Hélène DÉRY | Assistant, NDD |

# *Appendix 7*
# Acronyms

| | |
|---|---|
| ABET | Accreditation Board for Engineering and Technology |
| ANENT | Asian Network for Education in Nuclear Training |
| ANSTO | Australian Nuclear Science and Technology Organisation |
| BNEN | Belgian Nuclear higher Education Network |
| CEA | Alternative Energy and Atomic Energy Commission (*Commissariat à l'énergie atomique et aux énergies alternatives*) (France) |
| CFEN | *Conseil des formations pour l'énergie nucléaire* |
| CIEMAT | *Centro de Investigaciones Energéticas, Medioambientales y Tecnológicas* (Spain) |
| CIRTEN | *Consorzio Interuniversitario per la Ricerca Tecnologica Nucleare* (Italy) |
| CPD | Continuous professional development |
| CRL | Chalk River Laboratories (Canada) |
| CSN | Nuclear Regulatory Body (Spain) |
| DOE | Department of Energy (United States) |
| ECVET | European Credit system for Vocational Education and Training |
| EDF | *Électricité de France* |
| EHRO-N | European Human Resource Observatory Nuclear |
| ENEF | European Nuclear Forum (EC) |
| ENELA | European Nuclear Energy Leadership Academy |
| ENEN | European Nuclear Education Network (EU) |
| EN3S | European Nuclear Safety and Security School |
| E&T | Education and training |
| EU | European Union |
| FINNEN | Finnish Nuclear Education Network |
| HQP | Highly qualified personnel |
| HRD | Human resource development |
| IAEA | International Atomic Energy Agency |
| IEA | International Energy Agency |
| I2EN | International Institute for Nuclear Energy |

| | |
|---|---|
| **INPO** | Institute of Nuclear Power Operations |
| **INSTN** | National Institute for Nuclear Science and Technology (France) |
| **IPCC** | Intergovernmental Panel on Climate Change |
| **IRSN** | *Institut de radioprotection et de sûreté nucléaire* (Institute for Radiation Protection and Nuclear Safety) France |
| **JAEA** | Japan Atomic Energy Agency |
| **JNEN** | Japan Nuclear Education Network |
| **KAERI** | Korea Atomic Energy Research Institute |
| **KHNP** | Korea Hydro & Nuclear Power |
| **KINS** | Korea Institute for Nuclear Safety |
| **MEST** | Ministry of Education, Science and Technology (Korea) |
| **MKE** | Ministry of Knowledge and Economy (Korea) |
| **NDC** | Committee for Technical and Economic Studies on Nuclear Energy Development and the Fuel Cycle |
| **NEA** | Nuclear Energy Agency |
| **NEI** | Nuclear Energy Institute |
| **NKM** | Nuclear Knowledge Management (IAEA) |
| **NPES** | Nuclear Power Engineering Section (IAEA) |
| **NPP** | Nuclear power plant |
| **NRC** | Nuclear Research Centre (United Kingdom) |
| **NRR** | Nuclear research reactors |
| **NSERC** | Natural Sciences and Engineering Research Council (Canada) |
| **NtUss** | Nuclear Technology Undergraduate Student Society (Korea) |
| **OECD** | Organisation for Economic Co-operation and Development |
| **PSI** | Paul Scherrer Institute (Switzerland) |
| **R&D** | Research and development |
| **RR** | Research reactor |
| **SNE-TP** | Sustainable Nuclear Energy Technology Platform (EC) |
| **THF** | Thermal-hydraulic facilities |
| **UNENE** | University Network of Excellence in Nuclear Engineering |
| **UOIT** | University of Ontario Institute of Technology (Canada) |
| **UPM** | *Universidad Politécnica de Madrid* |
| **US NRC** | Nuclear Regulatory Commission (United States) |
| **WNU** | World Nuclear University |


NUCLEAR EDUCATION AND TRAINING: FROM CONCERN TO CAPABILITY, ISBN 978-92-64-17637-9, © OECD 2012